shower power

shower power

by
HELEN FLEDER

Photographs by Neil Winokur

M. EVANS AND COMPANY, INC. / NEW YORK

M. Evans and Company, Inc.
216 East 49 Street
New York, New York 10017

Library of Congress Cataloging in Publication Data

Fleder, Helen.
    Shower power.

    1. Exercise for women.   2. Hydrotherapy. I. Title.
GV482.F57   613.7'045   78-9718
ISBN 0-87131-273-5

Design by Joel Schick

Manufactured in the United States of America

9 8 7 6 5 4 3 2 1

To
The gems in my life — my family.
To my adoring husband Bob; to John, Peggy and
Bob, and Richard, my dearest children; to Joel, my
grandson, and to my wonderful mother-in-law, Adel.
Their love, devotion, and pride have been an
inspiration in every creative endeavor.

Contents

Acknowledgments

I wish to thank:
Sis and Bette Ann Harris, whose expertise in
physical therapy guided me in the right
direction;
Dr. Marilyn Moffet, who was supportive and
encouraged the concept of this book;
Alison Bond, who helped shape the book;
Meredith Bernstein and Anita Goodman who
made it all possible.

Author's Note

Think of your body as the temple of the spirit: clean,
pure, healthy, and strong. Think that it is firm and
flexible; pure and clean as a crystal; fresh, soft
supple like a fresh blown flower.

Sachindra Kumar Majumdar,
from *Introduction to Yoga Principles
and Practices*

For the major part of my life, I have been involved with
body movement. In the field of dance, I have performed, taught,
and choreographed. I have used movement as therapy for the
blind, the retarded, and the emotionally disturbed. As an artist, I
find that most of my drawings and sculpture relate to movement
of the female body. I feel that movement is the universal
language of expression, freedom of movement the most precious
gift of all.

To help every woman maintain that freedom through flexibility is the underlying theme of this book.

H.F.

INTRODUCTION

Wet, Warm, and Wonderful

Today's woman is a pacesetter—a person who sets high standards for herself and is ever conscious of her image. She is basically an active person. She knows that the values of keeping fit are unquestionable. She knows that staying in shape is the best antiaging pill on the market and that regular exercise is the energizer that keeps her going! She can take exercise in small or large doses, but if she doesn't do it regularly, she realizes only too well that she is cheating herself and her

1

body of life's most precious gift—the look and feeling of youthful vitality, regardless of age.

Today's woman finds spare time a rarity. She is aiming for a more positive self-image and wants to maintain a trim figure, but is often frustrated because her day's myriad activities leave her with little time for exercising.

She also admits that exercise—with a capital E—can be a dreary bore! How often do we determinedly embark on a daily program of calisthenics only to lose our initial enthusiasm after a week or so. No one knows this better than I. Although ballet was my world for many years (as a student I studied with George Balanchine), with my children grown, I now devote most of my time to other creative art forms, and I have replaced dance with sculpting, working hours at a time with energy focused in an equally demanding but more sedentary fashion. It wasn't always convenient to maintain the discipline of daily exercise that I knew only too well was the key to staying in shape, and in time the inevitable happened: My back muscles rebelled from stress and strain and much neglect. Wielding a hammer and chisel was a poor substitute for whirling around in toe shoes!

Just like every other woman, I could never find the *ideal time* and *right environment* to carry through a daily exercise routine. It wasn't always convenient to find those few precious moments each day alone with my quiet thoughts in a place that was cozy, warm, and conducive to relaxing, stretching, and limbering up.

Then, not long ago, something exciting happened.

I had been to a physical therapist for treatment for my back, and before therapy, which took the form of back stretching, a hot, wet pack was placed directly on the muscles involved. It worked well and gave me an idea. Why not do my basic warm-up exercises at a time when there was wet heat directed on my back — as there was each time I took a shower?

This proved to be the magic elixir! I could enjoy the benefits of bathing *and* of exercising right there in my own shower or bath. I could feel the juices flowing as I began to limber up and take full advantage of the warm water on the back muscles. With my shower and bath providing the water, I designed a sequence of exercises that proved to be practical and effective. They worked like a charm!

It didn't take long to realize that I had in the bathroom the makings of my own private spa. This tranquil atmosphere provided the perfect place to shape up at my own pace and with as much privacy as I'd ever want. A few simple exercises under the kiss of a shower spray as it stimulated my blood circulation, or a series of stretches as I reclined in my soothing bath, and those tight muscles were ready for action.

The stretches that I did after my shower to complete the routine really proved to me the power of the shower. I could get an even better stretch, yet with less effort. What more could I ask for?

These exercises for the shower or bath proved to be amazingly effective for me. And they can be just as effective for you, too. Muscle warm-ups and the series of stretches that I designed are perfect for shaping you up *and* helping you maintain a trim, youthful figure. Whether you are a shower or a bath person—and it doesn't make any difference which—try them and notice their effect on your body. You'll be delighted with the results, especially when you realize how much more responsive your body is to movement.

You may be wondering just what kind of exercises can be done within the confines of a bathroom, or how safe it is to move about in the bathtub or shower. Let me explain.

The muscles warm-ups (or stretches) can be adequately and *safely* done in an area no wider or longer than the average bathtub. You'll find safety precautions included with the exercises in Chapter II. The exercises that follow your bath or shower are done while the muscles are still flexible. If the area in your bathroom is too small, just use any warm room nearby with a rug or carpet.

Maybe you are the kind of woman who already does exercises regularly—you work out in class, at a spa, or go to a gym? You may be a tennis or ski enthusiast, or perhaps the much envied all-round athlete. If so, the Shower Power exercises will enable you to do any bending, stretching, or twisting movements with greater ease and effectiveness. For they add a plus to your flexibility and prevent the unnecessary strains that can occur when muscles aren't prepared for action.

We are all aware of tensions in everyday living. We live in a highly competitive society and most of us have to deal with more than our share of stress and anxiety. This tension travels through the nervous system to the muscles in the back where they grab on and hold fast. If the tension remains too long, our muscles become rigid, and tight muscles can mean trouble. Some people have to deal with tight muscles as a genetic inheritance. I can vouch for that. For many years my lower back presented problems, but today, if I put too much strain on it, the message reaches me via the muscles and I can relieve it within a day or two by working out with my Shower Power routine. Fortunately, even in the fashion world the trend is for clothes that protect the muscles in cold, damp weather; leotards and tights, which used to be essentials in a dancer's wardrobe, have now become fashion items.

Whether it is tension, stress, or climate, our muscles need all the help they can get. Is it any wonder then that Shower Power is for you—

> The woman who wants to gain or keep a slim, youthful figure
>
> The professional person who has to withstand business pressure
>
> The homemaker who must cope with household tensions
>
> The worker who sits at a desk all day
>
> The adolescent as she developes lifelong patterns of posture and muscle use
>
> The person who finds it hard to get going in the morning because of stiffness
>
> The person who needs to unwind after a busy day
>
> The woman who participates in active sports and wants to prevent strain and injury.

You are probably in there somewhere! We all are.

Shower and bath time are part of every woman's routine, and morning or evening, Shower Power fits into the day's schedule as naturally as mealtime. It won't take long for you to appreciate the benefits of wet, warm, and wonderful workouts. Whether it is to loosen early morning stiffness from lying like a pretzel all night, or to prepare your muscles for daily activity, you'll find the combination of the warm water and exercise will provide round-the-clock benefits.

You'll have to admit that the bathroom is an ideal spot to look at yourself in the mirror, focus on your shape, and realize that it isn't necessarily age that turns a youthful figure into flab, and firmness into bulges, but more often, poor postural habits. Here is where the Shower Power routine comes to the rescue! Having prepared the muscles by relaxing and stretching them, you will be ready for the very first exercise, which will do more to improve your figure than you ever dared hope for. Good posture is something priceless. No one can give it to you, but when you achieve it, you're treating yourself to the nicest gift you could ever receive.

In this book I have used simple language to describe the body and its functions and have intentionally avoided anatomical terms that may be unfamiliar to the reader. All the comments on the exercises are strictly my own, based as they are on personal experience and a dancer's knowledge of body movement. The exercises that follow are all basic ones for women of any age. If you have any doubts or physical problems, you should of course check with your doctor before exercising.

Shower Power means water power that is wet, warm, and wonderful. When you are showering, the water is stimulating and invigorating. When you are reclining in it, the water is soothing and relaxing. Water has been used through the ages in hydrotherapy, as many doctors can testify.

Shower Power has worked wonders for me, and I know it can do the same for you. And once you discover how wonderfully it can work, I hope you will want to tell your family and friends about it. Never again will you let the benefits of bathing go down the drain!

shower power

1

Shower Power and Your Body

Did you know that

- Good natural posture is *the* best exercise for the figure because it's the only one you can do continuously and carry with you wherever you are?
- Good natural posture flattens the tummy, tightens the buttocks, and slims the waist?
- Good natural posture aligns the pelvis in correct position?

- Good natural posture improves your breathing, circulation, and the flexibility of your body?
- Good posture is the natural way to stretch and tone the muscles that determine your shape? And that daily stretching loosens tight back muscles?

Did you know that

- *One postural exercise can build enough muscle tone to flatten your tummy* — and do wonders for your body at the same time?

It's all possible because your abdominal muscles have "Memory Power" — when you activate them frequently enough, in time they will respond automatically.

Although every woman can have these benefits, maintaining good posture often eludes her because she believes it requires a great deal of effort with no guarantee of success. As you will soon discover, there is one wonderful exercise that will change your postural habits easily and naturally — and do wonders for your body at the same time. Shower Power prepares you for it by warming and stretching your muscles. One "Dynamic Exercise" insures it!

FORM

Before you begin to enjoy all the benefits of Shower Power exercises, though, let's think a little about your body in terms of form and movement. Next time you step into the bathroom, take a few moments alone to stand in front of your mirror—full length, if possible, with no clothes on. Pause for a moment to really look at your body. It belongs to you and there's no reason not to appreciate it or be proud of it. However, it reflects much of your attitude about yourself. You may fool anyone about the way you feel, but you can't fool your body!

Form Is Figure

A beautiful body does not necessarily mean a perfect figure. But it is a body that radiates self-assurance and moves eloquently with that certain something called style. It's a body that belongs to every woman who is *posture proud*, who thinks elegance rather than glamour. It's what makes a woman look regal even though she may be wearing rags. It gives stature to the petite woman just five feet tall and confers on any body a look of youth and vitality.

While good posture determines good form, it cannot be taken for granted. Most of us had good posture when we were young but neglected it when we weren't even aware we were doing so. In due time adverse postural habits formed—some muscles worked overtime, others hardly worked at all. The result? Midriff bulge!

As a dancer and artist, I see the body as a creative work of art. I think we observe our own body in a rather superficial way, wishing we were taller—or slimmer—or sexier. Or we think of shape when we should be thinking of carriage. We forget one thing: how beautiful and well-designed an instrument the body really is, deserving of our optimum effort to keep it tuned and conditioned!

Figure Is Posture

Tall and thin may be beautiful for high-fashion models, but it certainly doesn't have to be the standard for most women. Your shape is influenced by heredity, height, and bone structure; your weight by intake of food and the number of calories you burn. Don't let your old friend, the bathroom scale, fool you because it tells you how much you weigh. What you weigh isn't any more important than the way you carry that weight!

You've probably heard about posture and carriage from the time you first started school, when you were told to "stand up straight" or "hold in your stomach"—irritating phrases because you understood why but not how. What I can tell every woman is that there *is* a simple, foolproof way to develop and maintain good posture, and a system that is neither difficult to learn nor uncomfortable to do.

Before getting down to the specifics of the figure-posture story, it is useful to relate it to *your* body. And the simplest way of doing that is to *see* it happen to you, *feel* it happen. Then you can *believe* it and understand why it will work. As you read the following pages in this chapter, take the time to look at your own body in a mirror. You will find it most helpful.

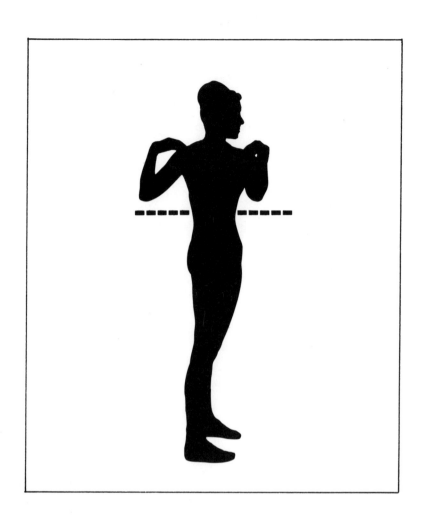

Posture Is Alignment

Correct posture and alignment of the spine are one and the same. They are the key to your good form. Look in the mirror and turn sideways to observe the shape of your spine in profile. Picture it as being made of attached sections or links. These links are called vertebrae and are supported and surrounded by muscles. Between the vertebrae are disks of cartilage that allow the spine to stretch, bend, and rotate; they provide suppleness. When the vertebrae are well-aligned, they link together like a chain and give the back mobility. Back muscles also have to work harmoniously in order to allow the body to move freely without strain, and so alignment and properly toned muscles are both essential.

If you look at your spine once more, you will notice that it is curved, not ramrod straight. Every back has a normal amount of curve. Some people have an accentuated curve. (If, when you lie down on the floor on your back with legs outstretched, you can slip one hand under the small of the back, above the buttocks or derrière then the chances are that you need to concentrate on pelvic adjustment.)

As a good illustration of perfect alignment in standing position, imagine there is a plumb line dropping down through the center of your body, as ear falls over shoulder, shoulder over hip, and hip over ankle.

But let's return to the word *alignment*. Look at yourself in the mirror, front view, and picture your body as being divided into two sections:

    a. neck, shoulders, and upper back (UPPER TORSO)
    b. pelvis, lower back (LOWER TORSO)

The dividing line is the waist. The position in which we hold our head and pelvis in relation to the natural curve of the spine is the key to perfect posture, a youthful well-shaped body, good muscle tone, and the degree to which we are able to move with ease and flexibility!

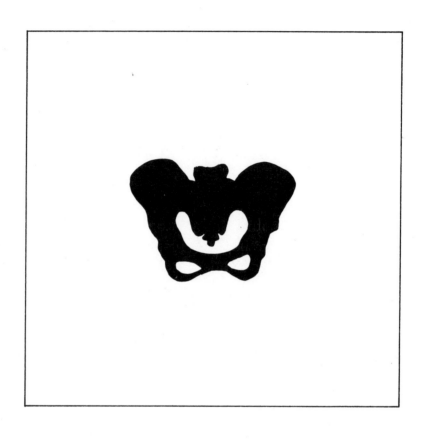

Alignment Means Adjustment

Surprisingly, most women do not stand with their pelvis in erect, correct position. This is partly because pelvic alignment is something few women are aware of, and partly because adjusting that alignment requires activating your abdominal muscles.

However, pelvic alignment is vitally important to every woman. Her pelvis was designed as a basin, a receptacle for housing the female organs. Her abdominal muscles support the weight of those organs by maintaining the pelvis in correct position. When muscles become weak and the pelvis tilts back out of position, the digestive organs sag, causing the only too common abdominal bulge. I've seen many weight-conscious women achieve slim figures and yet not be able to flatten their tummies!

Pelvic alignment involves tilting the pelvis. There are two sets of muscles that work together to tilt the pelvis into erect position and stabilize it so that alignment can be maintained. These muscles are located in the derrière and in the abdomen. The first exercise you'll learn will teach you how to maintain that pelvic tilt, a minor adjustment to your posture, a major change in your figure! Once your muscles are properly conditioned, you will find the adjustment coming far more easily and readily.

Adjustment Means Well-Conditioned Muscles

Making the pelvic adjustment depends on how well your muscles are able to respond. Well-toned muscles are normally elastic. The more you put them to work, the stronger and more flexible they become. When not in use (and the abdominal muscles are among the most neglected of all), they become lazy, lose their elasticity, and cause the flesh around them to become flabby. Conversely the more frequently you use them, the firmer they become.

Let's take a brief look at what the muscles do.

They act as the "hinges" to the separate parts of the body. They control movement. If the muscles are truly relaxed and are trim, they prepare the way to total fitness.

One of the ballet dancer's admired qualities is her long graceful look, the way her head and torso form a harmonious line and give her body the appearance of seemingly endless elongation. She has learned to achieve this by strengthening muscles in her abdominals and in her back. It is the reason she has a flat tummy and derrière, as well as a firm bosom. As it works for the dancer, so it can work for you. There's no magic to it!

There is one thing to be considered before you can reeducate your muscles to become strong, active, and lively so that they can do the job intended. Ask yourself whether they are relaxed or carrying any undue tension, for it does make quite a difference!

Back Muscles Need to Be Relaxed

The prime targets for tension, anxiety, fatigue, or prolonged inactivity are the muscles in your back, since tension grabs onto the neck, shoulders, and upper back areas. Every time I take an automobile trip and have to sit in the car for more than a few hours, my back muscles tighten like a drum. Picture it this way — the muscles respond to thoughts and actions like a switchboard. The message comes in loud and clear; the result is that as tension develops, muscles tighten, shorten, and lose elasticity. Is it any wonder that muscles need all the help they can get? What better reason for treating all the muscles in your body to wet, warm, and wonderful stretching?

Abdominal Muscles Need Firming

Once you have prepared your back muscles for bending and stretching, they will be ready to work to capacity. The star of Shower Power is the Dynamic Exercise, for it tones and strengthens the muscles that determine our posture. The exercise itself involves muscle contraction, and here's what that means. A strong muscle is firm, hard, and flexible; it has developed tone. When the muscle contracts and is held in contraction for a few seconds, it works to full capacity in static tension. Since you are aiming to strengthen the derrière and the abdominal muscles, you'll be using this tension in a *pinch-pull* action. Each time you do it, you'll be firming and strengthening those muscles as well as tilting the pelvis into an aligned position.

Let's begin with just a pinch action. Try doing it first in front of a mirror. Stand up and cup your hands around your derrière. *Pinch* the muscles of the derrière together, squeezing them as hard as possible. Hold the squeeze for about eight seconds. Feel the tightening of those muscles? Now relax and let go. As you pinched you tightened and contracted the derrière muscles in a *hold* or *isometric* contraction. Remember the feeling—you'll soon have it again as you do the first exercise.

MOVEMENT

What correct alignment is to a woman's form, relaxed but controlled movement is to effective exercising. Shower Power focuses on the *quality* rather than the quantity of exercises. It concentrates on exercises that can easily be done in a confined area. To get maximum results from these exercises, it would help to reduce movement to its basic elements and consider two important catalysts—isolating upper torso from lower torso whenever possible and using rhythmic breathing whenever beneficial. Let's begin with isolation.

Isolating the Torso

Suppleness means a limber spine that can move freely without stiffness, allowing the body to bend, twist, turn, and stretch.

Since your spine is flexible, it enables the upper back and rib cage to move independently from the lower back. The center, where your waist is, becomes the pivotal point. (For your shower exercises particularly, it is important to be aware of the lift of the rib cage, allowing for maximum stretchability of the spine.)

Most of the Shower Power exercises focus on either the upper or lower back, moving one part independently of the other. The degree to which you are really achieving flexibility depends on which muscle groups perform the work and is the prime factor in what "isolation" of movement is all about. Here is a good example. As you stand in front of the bathroom mirror, twist your torso so that it turns to the right, then return to neutral position. Repeat again and notice whether your hips and legs moved around at the same time. Now imagine that you were a puppet moving only when strings were pulled. If the strings were attached to the top of your shoulders, pulling only the shoulders and upper back to the right, you would twist without any movement from the waist down. You would, in a word, "isolate" the muscle movement, keeping it within the rib cage or upper torso. I will be using the puppet image in some of the exercises that follow to help you feel where the action is and bring the essential muscle groups into play.

Rhythmic Breathing

Rhythmic breathing provides a very natural way of bending the body without strain. The reason for this isn't hard to follow. If muscles are tight, they are short; when they are relaxed, they lengthen. If you are aiming for a good deep bending stretch it makes sense to do it when the muscles in the back are long and supple. And rhythmic breathing can help those muscles to relax. Rhythmic breathing is not quite the kind of breathing you do normally. It is a slower, deeper, more fluid type of breathing in one steady stream that fills the lungs with oxygen and the body with vital energy. Rhythmic breathing is not only beneficial to body conditioning, but to spine flexibility as well. It is an exercise in itself, so it takes a little practice before it feels naturally comfortable. Just as every body has its own rhythm, so the tempo of rhythmic breathing is individual. Take it at your own pace and practice it a few times.

Here's how you begin:
   1. Breathe in through the nose (this is important), as though you were smelling the delicious fragrance of a flower or your favorite perfume. Breathe s-l-o-w-l-y and s-t-e-a-d-i-l-y!
   2. B-L-O-W out through the mouth as slowly and steadily as you breathed in, as though you were gently blowing soap bubbles into the air. In a seated position, repeat the breathing several times, and try it with your eyes closed. You will release energy and tension with each breath. The more you relax the more you will be able to breathe fluidly—and that's what it's all about. Aim to extend the rhythmic breathing for as long as you comfortably can. I would suggest you begin with a count of six each time you inhale and each time you exhale, then increase to about ten to twelve. As you

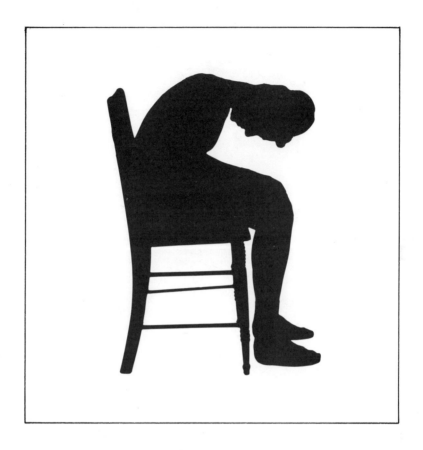

combine rhythmic breathing with the exercises that follow, remember that *breathing in* prepares for the movement, revitalizing the body; *breathing out* allows for the movement, relaxing the muscles for ease and flexibility.

To prove how well it can work for you, here is an example. Drop your head forward, letting it hang down as far as possible. Notice some tightness now in the muscles in the neck, for they control how far down

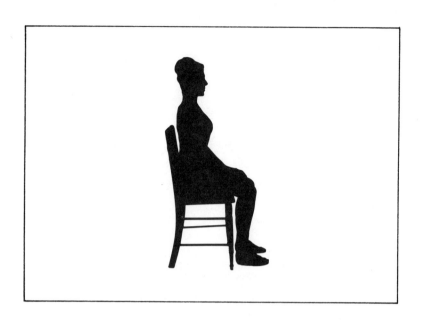

the head drops. Raise your head to its normal position. Now repeat this using rhythmic breathing. Breathe in slowly and deeply through the nose. This time let the head drop forward as you breathe out, again as though blowing gentle bubbles, in one continual breath, for as long as possible. You will notice how much farther down your head has dropped as the muscles in your neck relaxed, allowing for greater flexibility. Here's one way to look at it—when it comes to tension, breathing is relieving.

If this didn't work too easily the first time, don't be discouraged. Try a few more times until you are relaxed enough that it happens. When you consider how long you may have been holding on to any tightness, you shouldn't be too surprised that it takes time to let go of it! I think you will realize too that as your head drops forward, you are stretching the spine—a major focus of Shower Power exercising.

The Dynamic Posture Exercise

The Dynamic Exercise, which I referred to before as the star of Shower Power, is the most important exercise in the whole program because it combines relaxation, alignment, stretching, toning, and breathing, Once you have learned it, you will understand how inter-related with all the other exercises it is. You can practice the exercise as I describe it here, but when you repeat it immediately after your bath or shower stretches, you will notice a difference, for the bath and shower stretches all prepare your muscles for the Dynamic Exercise. Since many women have tight back muscles, any adjustment they try to make by correcting poor postural habits may seem difficult at first. So shower and bath exercises will prove to be a blessing, as you will soon discover—the warmth of the water will help your muscles respond and the more responsive your muscles, the easier you can adjust them.

Repeated faithfully, the Dynamic Exercise is the one exercise that does everything for your figure. Equally important, it elongates the spine and strengthens and protects vulnerable back muscles.

You will learn it first as a two-part exercise: the pinch-pull-hold isometric to align the pelvis and a roll-up stretch to align the head. Take it step-by-step and you'll see how basic and simple good posture really is.

Although you will be repeating your Dynamic Exercise when standing, the best way to learn it is from a supine position.

PART 1 - DYNAMIC EXERCISE - "PINCH-PULL-HOLD"

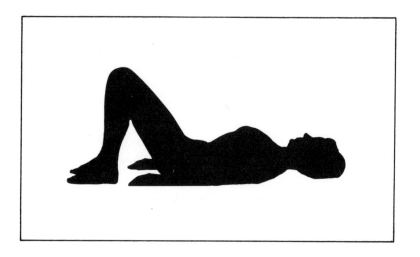

Supine Pelvic Tilt

For: Aligning the pelvis; toning the derrière muscles; strengthening the abdominals; flattening the tummy

Where: On the bathroom or bedroom floor where there is a carpet or rug. What you are doing here is tightening up the muscles in the derrière and at the same time reaching the abdominals as you tilt the pelvis. The most effective way to learn this is to lie on your back. Here on the floor, without gravity's pull, you will find it easier to get the feel of contracting muscles.

Preparation: The best time to do this exercise is immediately following your shower or bath. Lie on your back in a relaxed position on the floor. Extend your arms, palms down, so they are in line with your hips; bend the knees in as close to your hips as possible, keeping the feet flat on the floor and shoulder-distance apart. Relax so that you feel the back of your neck and shoulders sinking into the floor. Make sure that your feet are completely parallel—knees shouldn't tilt inward. Keep your chin tucked in, and relax.

1. Breathe in slowly and fluidly, filling your lungs with as much oxygen as possible.
2. Breathe out just as slowly and, as you do, *pinch* the derrière together and *pull* the navel in toward the floor as though it were going down through your back. Feel the contraction of your abdominal muscles? That's fine!
3. Relax and rest a few moments.
4. Repeat the first two steps, but this time hold the contraction at least six to eight seconds and try to feel your derrière roll "under" and lift slightly off the floor.
5. Relax and let go.
6. Repeat the exercise, trying to achieve fluid, steady breathing, and building the abdominal contraction that will tilt your pelvis forward and at the same time flatten your back.
7. Repeat several more times as you pinch-pull-hold.

Helpful Hints: Thinking of the puppet will prove a great help when you try this exercise. Let's pretend there is a string attached to your navel. As you pull back the navel, feel as though the string were being pulled through the small of your back into the floor. I hope this image will help you get the derrière and abdominal muscles working to their maximum. It may not happen right away, so keep with it! Be patient and work at it. You'll find the fluid breathing most helpful too. Each time you exhale, the muscles in your back relax and become more elastic, allowing the pelvis to tilt and the back to elongate.

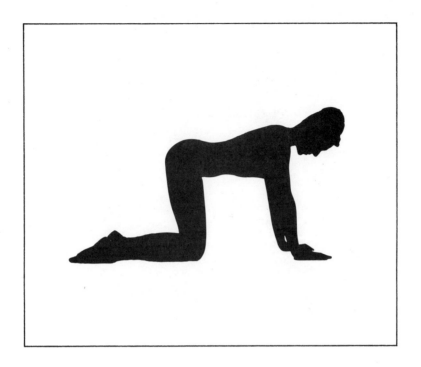

Kneeling Pelvic Tilt

If you have never done the Pelvic Tilt before, or feel a bit stiff in your back as you do it, here is a good way to practice the exercise so that you can loosen any tight muscles. Instead of holding the contraction, this Pelvic Tilt is done as one smooth movement—one continual rolling motion. Kneel on the floor on all fours, keeping your arms straight. Relax your back and let your head drop down. Repeat the pinch-pull action slowly tilting the pelvis back and forth in one fluid movement as you breathe normally.

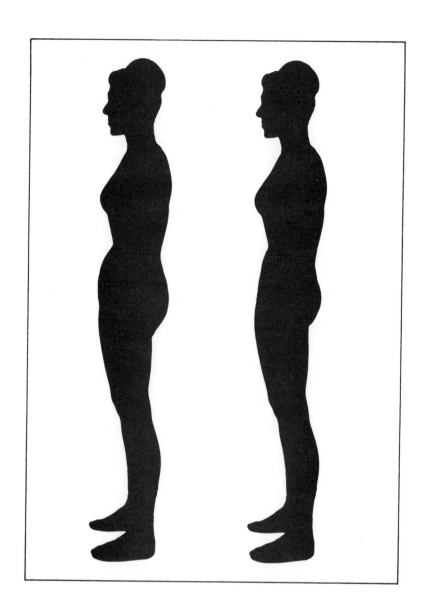

Standing Pelvic Tilt

Since you will be repeating the Pelvic Tilt as a postural exercise, it's important to get the feeling of doing it from a standing position. First try it with one foot up on a stool, the toilet seat, or the rim of the tub (bending one knee relaxes the lower back). Now try it holding on to any firm surface such as the basin or towel bar, repeating the exercise first as an isometric pinch-pull-hold, then in one continual movement as you breathe normally. This is the Pelvic Roll shower exercise. As you repeat pinch-pull-hold, remember the puppet image and think of a string attached to your navel. Try to feel the sensation of the string *pulling* the navel in toward the back. It is really quite a simple movement and you should think of its achieving two good things simultaneously: "pinching together" the derrière muscles and "pulling back" the abdominals. The results are firmer muscles in the derrière, an aligned lower back, and working abdominal muscles—the key to a figure a woman can be proud of. If you will conscientiously repeat the pinch-pull-hold movement once or twice every hour on the hour, you will begin to develop abdominal tone in a month's time. Don't get discouraged, stay with it, and you'll be amazed at the results. (Chapter III includes a more extensive *Supine Pelvic Tilt* as an après bath exercise. Once you have become comfortable with the pinch-pull action of the preceding exercise, the après bath stretch will be easy to learn.)

Now you are ready for the second part of the Dynamic Exercise.

PART 2 - DYNAMIC EXERCISE - "ELONGATE"

The second part of the Dynamic Exercise is really an adjustment of your upper back alignment. Here I will describe it as an exercise, but once you understand it you will easily be able to do it with a simple movement of the head. The Roll-Up/Stretch straightens and elongates the upper back and neck and aligns the head without tensing your shoulders or affecting the normal breathing pattern. We all get a bit sloppy and give in to gravity at times. Often we project our head forward, putting pressure on the neck muscles. Eventually this causes a round back and can add years to a woman's appearance. Fatigue, anxieties, and desk sitting can also cause this when you are least aware it is happening. How many of us are aware of our head and upper back posture? As we look at ourselves in a mirror, we automatically raise our head and therefore straighten our upper back, but when we walk away from the mirror we assume our *normal posture*, which too often means round shoulders and back!

Unfortunately it isn't easy to break old habits. If you were to lift your head in an attempt to straighten your back, you might inadvertently lift your shoulders or arch your back. The second half of the Dynamic Exercise shows you how to straighten up in a natural, relaxed way that will get lazy, tight muscles working. *Hint:* Once again, although you will be *repeating* the Roll-Up/Stretch from a standing position, learn it first while you sit relaxing. Once you've learned it, practice it, if possible, in the bath. There you can close your eyes, let go of mental tension, and include rhythmic breathing to induce total relaxation.

Roll-Up Stretch

For: Aligning and elongating the upper spine; proper head placement; stretching the neck muscles.

Where: In a sitting position in the bathroom or bedroom.

This does for the upper back what the Pelvic Tilt does for the lower back. It is simple and it works. If you do this exercise daily, you will be taking an important step toward correct head placement so vital for an erect spine.

Preparation: Sit in a chair, hands resting on the lap,

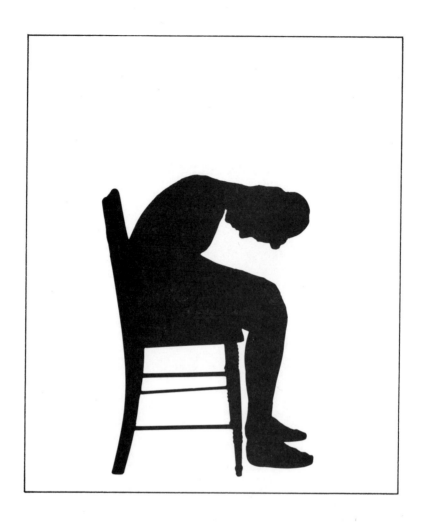

feet slightly apart on the ground. Relax your upper torso, leaning slightly forward, consciously letting go of
all tension in the neck and shoulders.

1. Breathe in slowly and deeply as you begin to roll
up the back one section at a time . . . first in the middle . . . then the upper back . . . lengthening the spine
as you go. Finally, lift the head until it faces forward,
ears in line with your shoulders and chin tucked in
slightly. That's the feeling to remember!

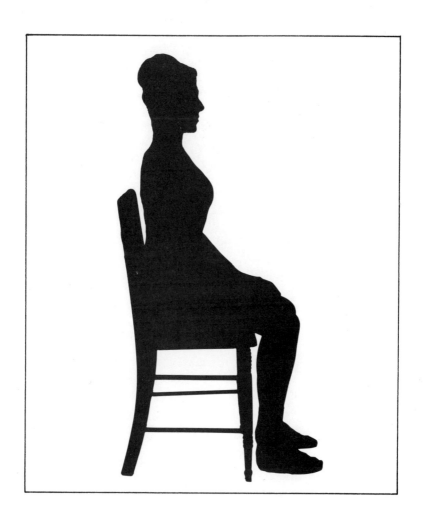

2. Slowly B-L-O-W out as you drop the chin down again, letting the head and shoulders relax completely as the upper back rolls down again.

3. Synchronize the breathing with the roll-up-roll-down movement. Repeat three more times.

4. Repeat the whole exercise from a standing position. Try it first with rhythmic breathing, then repeat breathing normally until you can elongate your back and align your head in *one fluid movement*.

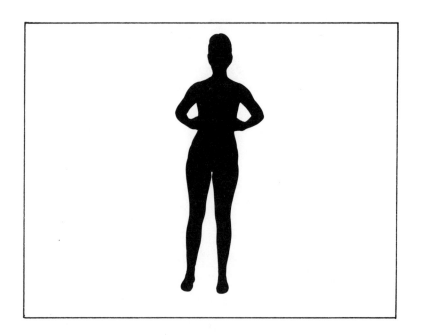

Helpful Hint: When combining rhythmic breathing with the Roll Up-Stretch, you can feel the action in your rib cage, as well as in your back. Repeat the exercise placing your hands directly on your ribs under your breasts. As you breathe in, feel the rib cage lifting up and spreading out, breathe out, relax, and feel the ribs drop down. As the rib cage lifts, it opens out like a balloon expanding and filling with air. If you were to put a tape measure around your rib cage, right under the bosom, you would see how many inches it had expanded! This feeling of *expanding* the rib cage *while you are breathing normally* is important to remember, as that is what you should do each time you elongate the back. One other point: There is hardly any perceptible movement in the shoulders as you breathe in; it is only the ribs that lift up and open. Chest heaving and shoulder lifting are absolutely no substitutes for proper deep breathing.

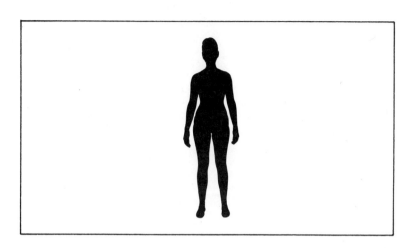

Dynamic Posture - Pinch-Pull-Elongate

Practice Supine Pelvic Tilt and Sitting Roll-Up Stretch many times until you feel comfortable doing them. When you are ready to combine them in standing position, don't consciously think about a breathing pattern, but concentrate on the feeling of good natural posture as you pinch-pull-elongate in one fluid movement. Begin with feet shoulder-distance apart, toes pointing forward, knees flexed. Relax your head, allowing it to drop down slightly. Then, as you pinch and pull, slowly elongate the back as you roll up into correct alignment. The more you practice the exercise, the stronger your muscles become, and with Memory

Power, eventually these muscles will respond without thinking and the Dynamic Exercise will become Dynamic Posture. Then you can relax and enjoy the way you look. Everyone else will, too!

Now that you are ready to begin Shower Power exercising, think of your body in terms of its form and movement, and try to remember the three R's of Shower Power:

RELAX the muscles with warm water and rhythmic breathing

RESHAPE your figure as you align with the Dynamic Exercise

REVITALIZE your energy by stretching and toning at your own pace, in the quiet tranquil atmosphere of the bathroom.

Once those postural muscles have relaxed, you can feel confident that with a bit of weight watching you can soon say goodbye to the midriff bulge and that out-of-shape stomach that even active sports won't take care of. "Pinch-pull-elongate" *will* work, *dramatically*—and it's all part of Shower Power. Shower Power is water power, yours to enjoy and benefit from, whenever you're ready!

Now it's time to take Dynamic Posture into your shower or bath where you'll feel the flow of each movement as fluid as the running water itself. Shower Power will help you discover how good it makes you feel to stretch when your muscles are rarin' to go—how deliciously supple and recharged with energy you will become.

2

The Private Spa

You're now ready to try a workable program of exercises that are right for you and that will fit in comfortably with your life-style. Let me remind you of the three R's of conditioning—Relax with the warm water and breathing, Reshape by aligning, and Revitalize by stretching. The three R's are essential for helping you do the exercises effectively and without strain. Combined, they help spell fluidity of movement.

The first exercises you'll be learning are those for the shower and the bath. It won't make a bit of difference whether you are the type of person who enjoys the refreshing sensation of a wake-up shower or perhaps likes to luxuriate in a warm, soothing bath. In terms of exercise both work just as well for preparing the body and making it more supple. So depending on your preference for a bath or a shower, choose from the exercise series that seems right for you. Either one will do much to improve your figure and condition your body, so it's up to you personally to tailor your routine to suit your needs and the demands on your time. Just remember: Stay with your exercise routine whatever you choose!

Shower and bath are particularly beneficial for upper back muscles. Since they stimulate blood circulation and release undue tension, these exercises prepare the body for stretching and enable the muscles to respond easily to daily activity. They are, in a word, relaxers. The shower exercises affect the upper back muscles in particular, while those in the bath focus mainly on muscles in the lower back and legs. The towel exercises in Chapter III—which you'll get to afterward— stretch the muscles in the torso and limbs by moving the joints through a full range of movement. As a complete head-to-toe workout, the towel exercises are good preparation for any daily activity whether you're sitting at a desk, running a household, or standing on your feet all day.

The remaining après shower and bath exercises focus on specific areas where stretching *and* toning are important. Some are isometrics, others are designed to utilize the resources in the bathroom or bedroom. Whatever you decide to do for yourself, remember that all these exercises are intended for people of any age. But use good judgment before doing them. If you have reason to question whether they are suitable for you, discuss the matter with your doctor.

Many of the exercises in this book are very flexible. Some shower stretches are equally effective from seated bath position. Many of the special exercises are ideal for shower, or bath. Follow the key along side each exercise as a guide. ▬▬ ▼

A word before you actually begin:

1. Read through all the exercises so that you understand what's involved, what you may need to have on hand.

2. Ease into the exercises a few at a time, taking each one slowly. Each exercise should seem comfortable to you before you add a new one to your repertoire. The series were designed to be done in sequence, so try them in the general order in which they appear.

3. Don't rush through them, and don't overdo an exercise—even if you think it's just marvelous! A little stretch goes a long way. Sometimes the harder you try, the more unnecessary stress you can build up in your neck or shoulders.

4. How long should you exercise? A practical program will take about twenty to thirty minutes once you've learned your exercises. The minimum is ten minutes; I find I do about twenty minutes each day.

5. Choose the time of day that's best for you. I would, however, recommend that you avoid strenuous exercise right before you go to bed, as it may be too stimulating. But whatever you do, do it regularly. It's the key to success!

6. Remember to include the rhythmic breathing pattern whenever indicated and to keep your movements fluid. Rhythmic breathing and fluid movements will help eliminate muscle strain and make stretching a good deal more comfortable.

IN THE SHOWER

The shower is fast becoming the environment where personal care begins. Massage sprays, French massage gloves, afterbath colognes, skin nourishing soaps and creams all help to make a woman feel good. But shower time is also prime time to think about your body in terms of shape. What better place to do this than here under the shower spray with the warm water pulsating down on your back.

Before beginning the exercises, here are some practical tips:

- Place a rubber mat (or rubber strips) on the floor of your shower or tub, for safer footing. You don't want to practice perfect alignment in a cast from hip to shoulder!
- Stand with your feet parallel and firmly planted on the mat, distributing your weight equally on both feet. Practice the shower exercises at least once before doing them under running water.
- Do the Dynamic Exercise as soon as you step out of the shower, repeating it several times.

- Make a conscious effort to relax, for this is the best place to literally drop all undue tension in the neck and shoulders.
- Keep a warm robe or bath towel on hand for drying, a towel for après bath series, as well as a warm—up suit to wear while exercising.
- If you want to, wear a plastic cap to protect your hair. You can't benefit from the warm water unless it's flowing directly onto your back. Some of the new shower heads allow you to adjust the spray to suit the exercise, so if you have one make use of it.
- Never close your eyes in the shower. And try not to breathe too deeply, for deep breathing can cause dizziness.
- If you have a narrow, stall shower you may have to adjust and turn slightly sideways to give yourself sufficient arm room.
- Before completing your shower routine, you may want to stand under cool water for a few seconds. Cool water is stimulating to the circulation and it closes the pores.

As you do your exercises, be sure that
- The shower head is focused appropriately (make use of a pulsating shower spray if you have one)
- You're thinking pinch and pull
- You're concentrating on fluid movement.

Shower Power is all yours! Let the warm water work wonders for you.

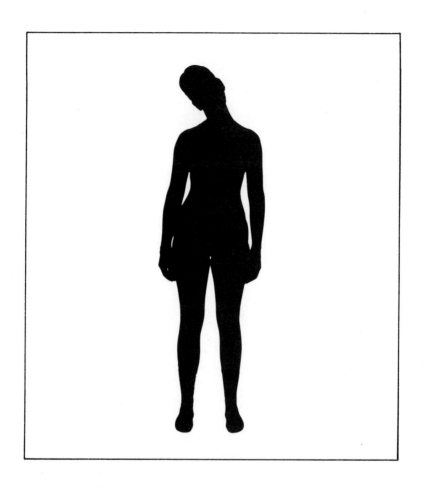

▬ Head Tilt

For: Stretching the neck muscles

This is one exercise where relaxation is the key—so let go of *all* that tension you may feel in the neck and shoulders. In the morning, this and the exercise that follows work particularly well to relieve any tightness from cramped sleeping positions.

Preparation: Stand up and focus the shower directly

onto your neck. Remember to keep the shoulders relaxed and down—and chin tucked in slightly.

1. Facing forward and looking straight ahead, slowly and gently drop your head to the right and feel your right ear reaching for the shoulder.

2. Slowly raise the head to an erect position.

3. Repeat this movement to the left, again with the feeling that the ear is reaching for the shoulder.

4. Continue tilting your head from right to left, repeating the whole movement four to six times. The more you relax, the greater the tilt, and the better the stretch.

Helpful Hint: Keep the movement slow, steady, and fluid—it's similar to a metronome.

▬▬ Head Rotations

For: Stretching the neck muscles

This is similar in purpose to the previous exercise and just as effective! Try combining them into one exercise.

Preparation: Stand with head erect and look directly in front of you.

1. Imagine that you have a piece of chalk attached to the end of your nose; draw two ovals slowly in the air with it. Start with a clockwise motion first.

2. Repeat, drawing two counterclockwise ovals this time.

3. Repeat both movements several times.

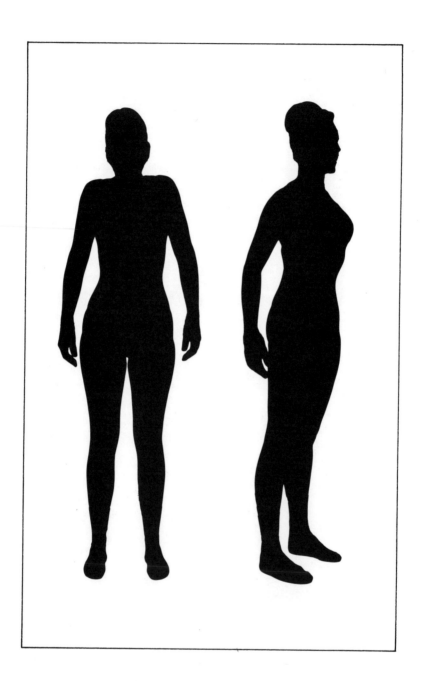

Shoulder Rotations

For: Loosening up the muscles in the shoulders and upper back

Treat yourself gently and begin by doing this exercise in slow motion, then increase the range of the circle somewhat. The shower spray combined with the shoulder action will give you a first-rate back massage.

Preparation: Stand up with your arms hanging loosely at your sides. Make sure that your chin is tucked in slightly and your shoulders are relaxed. Focus the shower spray on your upper back.

1. Lift your shoulders up and begin to circle them backward and downward, then forward and up, describing a continuous circle with them.

2. Begin with small circles, then gradually increase the radius of the circle until you feel the blood circulation stimulated as the upper back muscles loosen up.

Helpful Hint: Keep your head still! The movement should all be in the shoulders and upper back.

▰ Elbow Kiss

For: Stretching the upper back muscles; opening the rib cage

Now an exercise that is an excellent stretch for the upper back. The elbow kiss is an invigorating exercise, so don't hesitate to work at it—the warm water is just the right stimulant for this motion and will get your muscles stretched in no time! So enjoy it.

Preparation: Stand up and place your fingertips on your shoulders, keeping your elbows in close to the body. Focus the shower spray on the upper back.

1. Swing your elbows forward and in toward one another, trying to touch them.

2. Now swing them freely away from each other, back and apart. You'll feel the shoulder blades being pulled together as the rib cage opens. Drop the elbows close into the body and relax a few seconds.

3. Repeat these two movements, swinging the elbows forward and back.

4. Continue swinging four or five more times as you feel the marvelous expansion of the rib cage.

Helpful Hint: When this movement seems comfortable, try the next exercise—you'll need a little more room for Angel Wings, but the two exercises blend as one marvelous warm up!

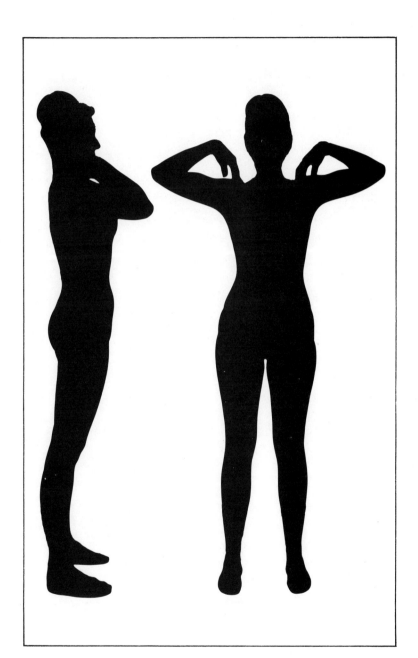

▬ Angel Wings

For: Loosening and stretching the muscles in the shoulders and upper back

I am particularly fond of this exercise because it works into the muscles in the upper back and at the same time will give you the marvelous feeling of expanding your rib cage. Let the movement flow as your arms swing out, then feel as though you could take off and fly! You will need maximum elbow room for this, so you may have to adjust your stance. If it isn't possible to do this in the shower try it as an après shower exercise.

Preparation: Stand up and place your fingertips on your shoulders and tuck your elbows into your sides. Keep your shoulders relaxed throughout.

1. Swing the elbows forward until they are at shoulder level.
2. Swing them down and then out to the sides, again to shoulder level. (Shoulders lift as elbows swing out)
3. Swing them down and forward, and then away from the body, describing two complete circles. End in the neutral position, ready to begin again.
4. Repeat these three movements — swing forward, sideways, circle and circle — at least three more times.

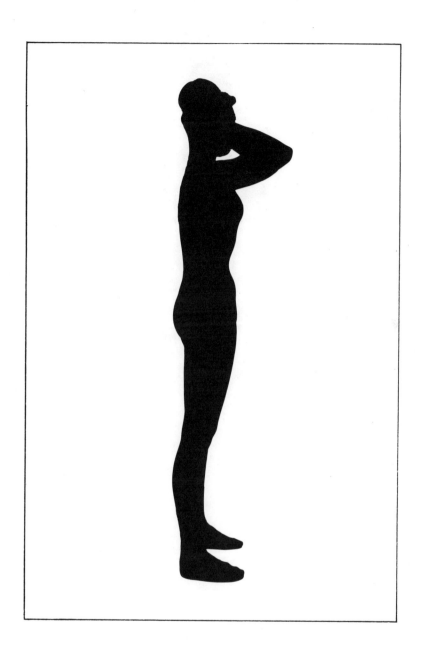

Helpful Hints: The more relaxed you are in the neck and shoulders, the easier it will be to swing your arms. The larger the circles you can describe, the more the

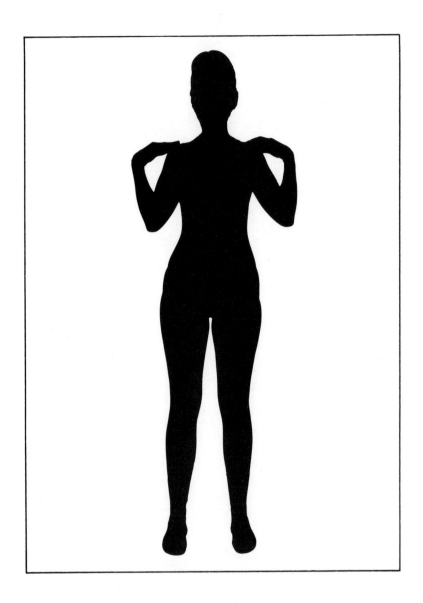

exercise works for the upper back muscles. Try to do this exercise as rhythmically as possible. It's really all one fluid motion.

If you want to add a neck stretch, you can include the following head movement. Repeat the whole exer-

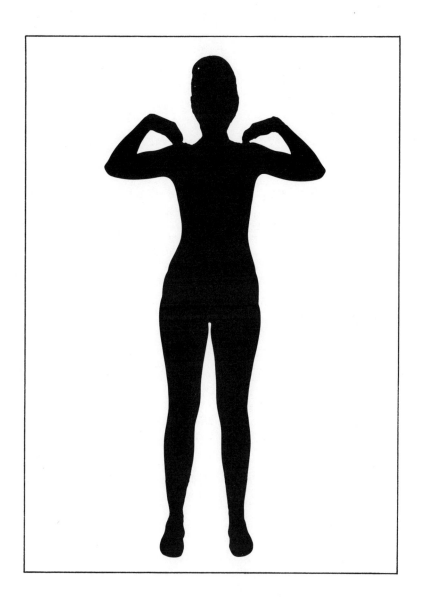

cise with these additions to each of the first three steps:

1. Drop the head down.
2. Lift up the head toward the ceiling.
3. Relax head and face straight ahead.

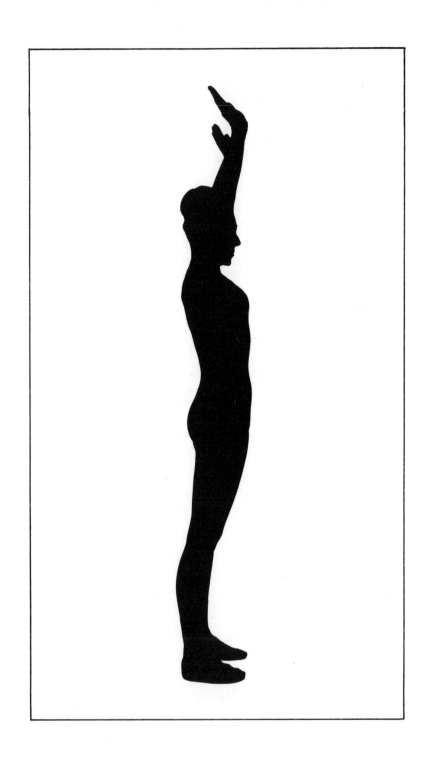

▰▰ Overhead Stretch

For: Strengthening the arms and upper back

Here's a wonderful stretch. You can think of elongation as well as alignment—they're both important.

Preparation: Stand up tall, bend the arms, and tuck the elbows in to the sides, with wrists flexed and palms up. Keep those abdominals pulled in tight for this one. Focus the spray on the upper back.

1. Facing forward, lead with the butt of the hands, pushing the hands up strongly toward the ceiling and continue pushing until the elbows straighten.

2. Turn your palms to face you, cupping the hands. As though you were "resisting," pull hard as you bring your arms down again. Relax a moment.

3. Repeat the pushing up-pulling down three more times.

Helpful Hint: To increase the strengthening of the arm muscles, place a washcloth in both hands; squeeze it firmly as you do this exercise from the beginning.

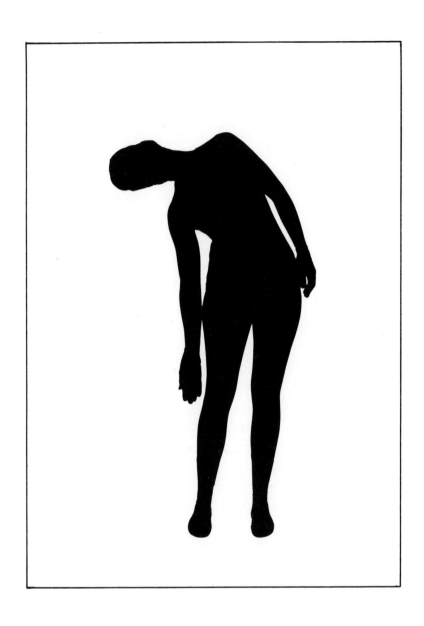

▬ Side-to-Side Bend

For: Stretching the muscles down the sides of the tor-so; slimming the waistline

It is vital when doing this exercise to keep the shoulders, hips, and ankles in one line. It's the whole secret of success in how to do this because shoulder, hip, and ankle alignment keeps the body from twisting (as opposed to bending) and maintaips correct body alignment. It's not how far down you go that gives you the proper stretch, but how you bend.

Preparation: Check alignment, moving from the shower spray, so that your head is erect. Eyes should be looking directly ahead. Focus the spray on the upper or middle back. Concentrate on relaxing your head, arms, and shoulders.

1. Drop your head down to the right (as for the Head Tilt, Chapter 2); now continue dropping a bit farther to the right, letting the right shoulder drop, and the hand slide down the leg. Try to go down as far as possible without straining.
2. Lift up and raise the head to its normal position.
3. Repeat the bend to the other side, bending the head to the left; then lift up.
4. Continue this dropping down-lifting up two or three times.

Helpful Hints: Dropping from right to left is one continuous movement, your head, shoulders, and arms bending from side to side. Here again it's like a metronome. The head starts each movement to the side.

Waist Twist

For: Loosening the middle back muscles; slimming the waist

This is yet another waist stretch—an exercise that, by twisting the upper torso, does so much for eliminating flabbiness.

Preparation: Stand slightly away from the shower, as in the previous exercise. Plant the feet firmly on the rubber mat, as though glued there, and relax the knees. Place the fingertips on the shoulders, tucking the elbows in to the sides. Focus the spray on the upper and middle back. Make sure the eyes are focused directly ahead throughout this exercise.

1. Swing the upper torso from the waist as far as you can to the right; now swing all the way through to the left, keeping your head facing forward.

2. Repeat the whole movement doing six to eight swings, moving shoulder and upper back only.

Helpful Hints: As I've mentioned before, there is a natural tendency to move your hips as you turn. Just remember that you *can* move the rib cage without moving the pelvic area (and now's the time to practice that), provided you keep the back elongated. That's what isolating the torso is all about.

Remember that this exercise is a free-flowing swing from right to left—and it really loosens up that upper back!

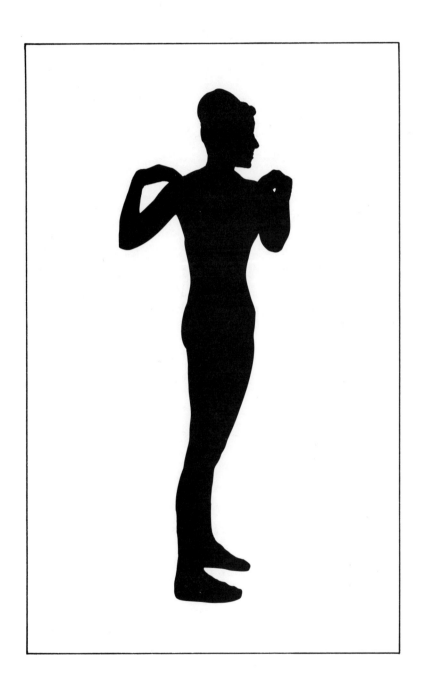

Pelvic Roll

For: Tightening of the derrière; loosening the muscles in the lower back

Here in the shower is the ideal place to practice the Pelvic Roll. With the warm water running directly onto those lower back muscles, the pelvis will move fluidly. This time, unlike during the Dynamic Exercise, you are *not* holding the muscles in contraction, but moving the pelvis fluidly as in the Kneeling Pelvic Tilt.

Preparation: Stand up and check your alignment. Make sure the knees are flexed and remain so during the exercise. Focus the spray on the lower back.

1. Gently pinch the derrière together and contract the abdominals until the pelvis tilts. Make sure your upper legs do not push forward as you tilt.

2. Release and let the pelvis move back again.

3. Repeat these two movements six times, tilting the pelvis quite slowly and fluidly so that you make it one continuous rolling movement.

Hip Rotations

For: Loosening the lower back muscles and pelvis

If you've ever watched someone with a Hoola Hoop, then you'll know what this exercise looks like. Children do it easily because their muscles are relaxed; with warm water on your back, yours can be too.

Preparation: Stand up with your feet placed firmly on the mat. Check to make sure your feet are parallel and shoulder-width apart. Focus the shower spray on your lower back.

1. Placing your hands firmly on your hips to stabilize them, swing the hips gently to the right and continue in a clockwise circle.
2. Continue circling them four times.
3. Reverse directions and now circle to the left.
4. Repeat both circles again.

Helpful Hint: Let your pelvis do *all* the work! And that means as little movement as possible in the upper torso. It's easy to do with regular practice.

IN THE BATH

Taking a bath is like taking an instant vacation. Here you can soak away hassle and worry, pour in a few drops of oil to moisturize your skin—or dried herbs to soothe aching muscles—and lie back to enjoy some precious moments of tranquility. Is it any wonder that this is the perfect time to loosen and stretch the muscles when it is here that exercising becomes easier and more comfortable?

Since you don't have to cope with either gravity or balance, the bath is the ideal place to close your eyes, abandon all thoughts except those of total relaxation, practice rhythmic breathing, and concentrate on stretching and strengthening back and leg muscles.

I have selected a group of head-to-toe stretches that I consider most beneficial. Chapter IV includes some additional ones, specifically for the feet and ankles.

Bathtubs come in assorted sizes and shapes, so you may have to make a minor adjustment in body position for some of the exercises. If possible, lie far enough down in the tub so that you can brace one foot against the end. You may want to omit an exercise you do not feel comfortable with; if so, try doing it after your bath, sitting on a rug (but don't forget it altogether!).

Avoid exercising in a bathtub where there is neither a rubber mat nor rubber strips. An inflatable pillow, placed at the head of the tub, will add to your comfort in some exercises (but it's not essential).

Fill the tub no more than three-quarters full while you're exercising—a nose full of water is not conducive to rhythmic breathing!

Before beginning your warm-ups, take time for soaking—at least a minute or two. Your muscles will thank you for that later!

A Preexercise Thought

Relaxing in the bath is everything! Before beginning here's a suggestion for you.

Lie back in the water—it should be about up to your shoulders—and close your eyes. Feel as though your face were molded out of wax and the warm sun was pouring down onto it, melting the wax as your eyes, ears, nose, and mouth become softer . . . and softer!

(You'll find other instant relaxers in Chapter IV.)

Shoulder Rotations

For: Loosening and relaxing shoulder and upper back muscles

This is one of my favorite relaxers. It's as beneficial to the desk sitter as it is to a sculptor like myself who spends hours at a time doing strenuous work. It is especially effective in the bath because you can close your eyes and relax any tight feelings in the face.

Preparation: Lie back comfortably with your knees slightly bent. Place your arms at your sides with the palms facing in toward the thighs.

1. Gently lift the shoulders, pulling them up, back, down, and then forward to make one continuous circle.

2. Continue circling at least six to eight times.

3. Relax and rest a few seconds; then repeat.

Helpful Hints: This exercise may be repeated sitting upright in the tub. From this position you can work into larger shoulder circles and give your upper back an even deeper stretch. Remember to keep your head still and let the shoulders do all the work!

Head Rotations (Chapter 2) are very similar and can be done quite effectively from a sitting position in the tub—just close your eyes for deeper relaxation.

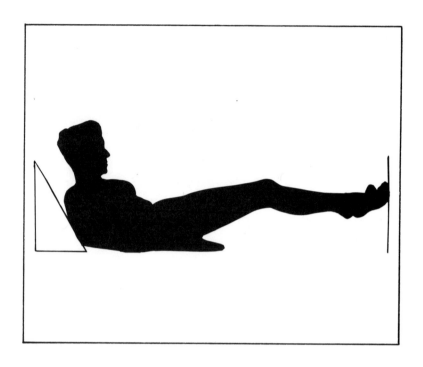

Pelvic Tilt

For: Relaxing the lower back muscles; tightening the muscles in the pelvis

The pinch-pull again, but with good reason! This time the warm water relaxes the back muscles, loosening the pelvis, allowing it to tilt easily. The legs brace the torso and really help you get a deep pinch-pull contraction. The bath position may seem less comfortable than the floor, but it still works well. Remember that each time you contract the muscles you are activating them, so to achieve toning the movements

66

must be slow. Bath time allows you the luxury for those few extra minutes, so there's no need to rush through this one!

Preparation: Lie back in the tub far enough so that your feet touch the end. Knees should be bent. (If you can reach the end of the tub with your feet, lift your heels up and press against the tub with the balls of your feet, using the tub as a brace.) Place arms at your side, palms down.

1. Pinch the derrière together and at the same time pull in your navel as though it were being sucked into the water.

2. Relax and release the contraction.

3. Repeat the pinch-pull action, but this time try to hold the contraction a few seconds longer, as you did in the Dynamic Exercise.

4. Repeat several times.

Helpful Hint: When the abdominals have developed tone—and that happens when you do this exercise regularly—you'll be able to feel your derrière lift up from the bottom of the tub, as the pelvis tilts forward. Then you'll know that you have reached those muscles that are the key to keeping your tummy and derrière firm.

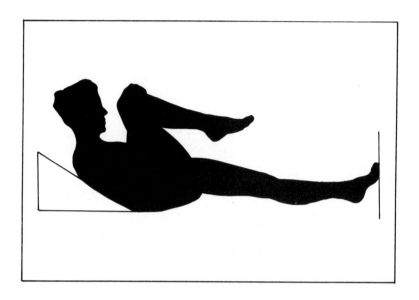

Knee and Ankle Hug

For: Loosening the muscles in the lower back

This is one of the best exercises I know to release strain in the lower back. It's a variation of the Knee Hug, which is probably familiar to you. Whenever my back tightens I do this exercise and find it most useful because it can be done from a sitting, standing, or lying position. Taking a bath is about as relaxing as you can get—and that relaxing feeling is well worth the time a bath takes.

Preparation: Lie back comfortably with your left leg stretched out and your right knee bent.

1. Place the right hand over the right knee and then the left hand over it, clasping the knee.

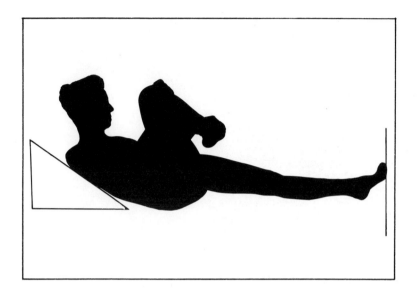

2. Slowly and gently, pull your knee in toward your chest. Continue to pull in about six or eight times, until your lower back muscles feel loose and flexible.

3. Remove the left hand from the knee and place it on your right ankle, gently pulling the ankle in as close to the groin as possible.

4. Now slowly and gently, holding onto both knee and ankle, pull the leg in toward the chest about six or eight times.

5. Stretch the right leg out and relax a minute. Then bend the left knee and repeat the whole exercise with the left leg.

Helpful Hint: The feeling of pulling in the leg should be similar to a rocking movement, as gentle as rocking a cradle.

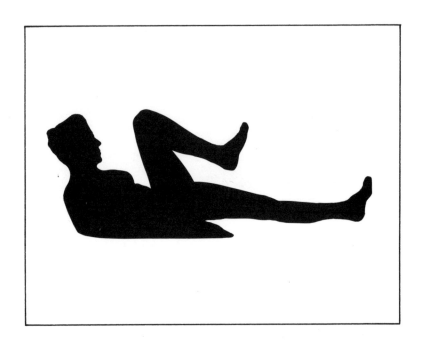

The Slapper

For: Loosening and stretching muscles in the lower back, legs, and ankles; strengthening the abdominals

This exercise works right into the lower back and helps to tighten the thighs at the same time. It may take a bit of practice, but the results are worth the trouble. Since it's a multipurpose exercise it is easier to learn in four stages; for a comfortable pace I'm suggesting a count for each stage. Once you become comfortable with this exercise, you'll appreciate how great it really is. We all tend to neglect warming up our feet and ankles. And this is a great way of combin-

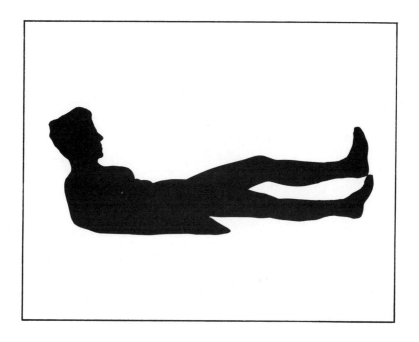

ing a muscle stretch with an exercise for joint flexibility; it flexes the feet and ankles while tightening the thighs.

Preparation: Lie back comfortably with arms at your sides, palms down. Bring the right knee in toward the chest, with the foot flexed (toe pointing toward the ceiling). Try placing the left foot up against the end of the tub for firmer support.

    1. With the heel leading, push your right foot forward until the leg is fully outstretched, skimming the surface of the water with your heel. (Count 1 and 2.)

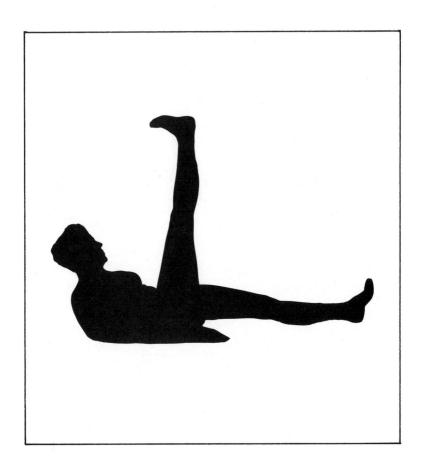

2. Pull in your abdominals, and as you do, lift the right leg up toward the ceiling as high as possible. Keep the foot flexed and the leg straight. (Count 3 and 4.)

3. Relax, and keeping the foot still flexed, bend the right knee toward you until the foot is just above the water level. (Count 5 and 6.)

4. Rotate the foot to the right, describing two

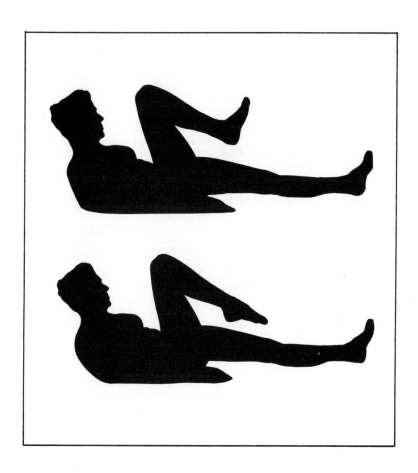

ovals; as you're rotating, make a real effort to slap the water with your toes as hard as possible. (Count 7 and 8.)

    5. Repeat once more, then place your leg down.

    6. Repeat the whole exercise with your left leg.

Helpful Hint: Repeat with rhytmic breathing. Breathe in with step 1—B-L-O-W out with step 2.

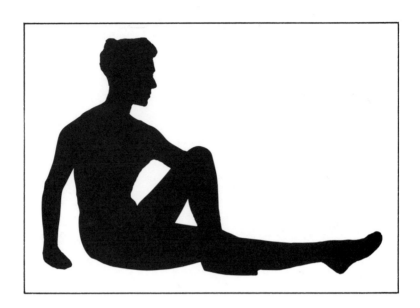

Torso Twist

For: Stretching the muscles in the middle back; elongating the back, torso flexibility.

All too often we get careless about posture and slump forward at times, shortening and tightening back muscles. Here you will be doing a torso twist to stretch the back muscles and keep the back flexible. And as you do, you'll correct bad postural habits which cause midriff bulges and thickening in the waist.

Preparation: Sit up close to the right side of the tub, extending the right leg. Bend your left leg and place it over the right one, pulling the left foot in as close to your body as possible, using the side of the tub as a brace. Elongate your back and pull in the abdominals.

1. Press your left elbow against the knee of the left leg, beginning to twist your upper torso to the right.

2. Continue twisting around to the right until you

74

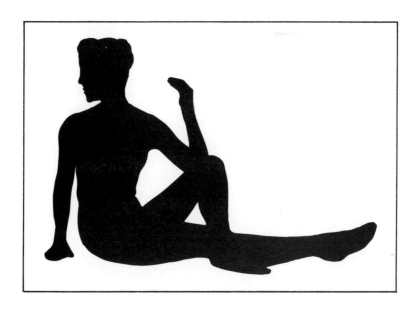

can place your right hand behind you, palm down, as a stabilizer.

3. Turn your head to the right and try to look directly behind. As you're twisting the head and upper torso as one piece, you'll feel the stretch from the top of the neck to the lower back. Once you've turned as far as possible, hold that position for a few seconds.

4. Relax. Breathe in and then as you B-L-O-W out, try to twist around just a *bit* farther.

5. Breathe in then out again, twisting even farther if you can. Untwist your torso, extend your left leg, and relax completely.

6. Now move a bit closer to the left side of the tub, pull in the right foot, and repeat the whole exercise to the left.

Helpful Hint: The rhythmic breathing pattern is very helpful here. Stretch. As you breathe out those muscles relax, allowing maximum movement in upper torso. The Result? A powerful and effective exercise!

Knee Bounce

For: Stretching the inner thigh

The inner thigh muscles are the first to get flabby yet often are the most neglected. Here's an easy way to get them stretched. In the bath this will take no extra effort at all! And by stretching the thighs you're working into the muscles of the pelvis as well. If you are cramped for space, adjust the position of your body by facing the side of the tub.

Preparation: Sit up tall with the left leg fully extended and the right leg bent so that the knee is parallel to the tub. Grasping the right leg at the ankle, place it on top of the thigh of the left leg. Put your left hand over the arch of your right foot and the right over the lower part of your right leg, stabilizing the leg as you hold it firmly.

1. Pull in the abdominals, and as you do so, press the right knee down as though it were reaching for the bottom of the tub.

2. Relax and let the right knee come up to neutral position.

3. Press the right knee down again, this time pressing and releasing it in a fast, continuous motion so that it feels as though you were bouncing the knee —with the accent down toward the bottom of the tub.

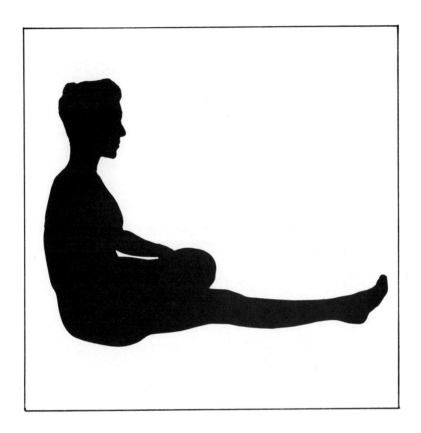

For a greater stretch, pull the ankle even closer toward you and continue bouncing.

4. Release the right leg and stretch it out.

5. Repeat the exercise, this time with the left leg bent.

Forward Bend

For: Stretching the lower back

I've found this a wonderful exercise for reaching into the lower back muscles. You have the end of the tub to hold on to, which will help give you an even greater stretch, so take full advantage of it.

Preparation: Sit up tall about an arm's length from the end of the tub and cross your legs. Keeping your arms parallel at shoulder height, bend forward and place your hands on the end of the tub. Look down at the water.

1. Drop your head and, bending the elbows, let the upper torso drop down toward the water.

2. Pull back, pushing against the tub end until your arms are straight again.

3. Continue dropping down-pulling back several times. The more you relax the elbows, the farther forward you'll be bending.

4. To add a hamstring stretch, sit farther back in the tub until you can straighten your legs. Brace your feet against the end of the tub. Grab onto your legs (as close to the ankles as possible) and repeat dropping down-pulling back action as in step 3.

Helpful Hints: To get the feel of sitting tall, imagine that a string attached to the top of your head was pulling you up toward the ceiling.

Repeat this exercise with rhythmic breathing: Breathe in as you pull back and blow out as you drop down. It's an added bonus if your back muscles are very tight.

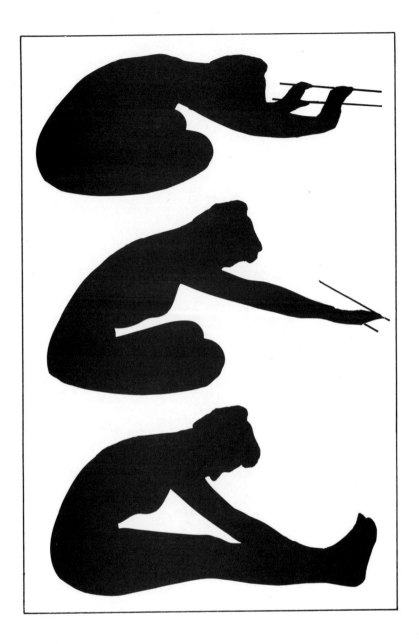

Each time you blow out think of blowing those bubbles and you'll be helping the back muscles to relax so that you can get a good stretch without strain! This exercise is a great warm-up for the towel stretches.

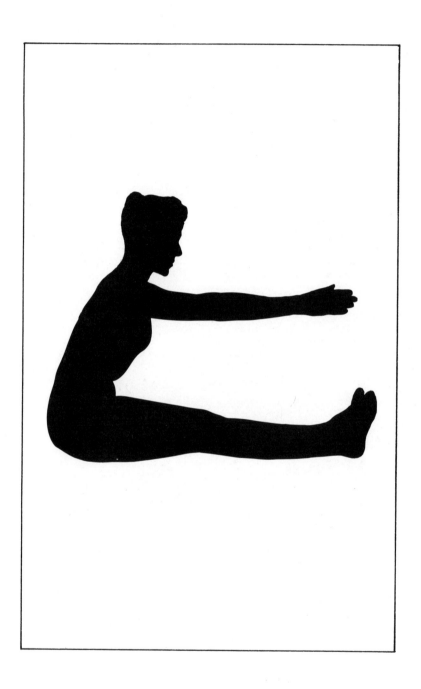

Forward Reach

For: Stretching the upper thigh and Achilles tendon
Here's another exercise where you can use the bath as a brace for the legs. So make the most of it!

Preparation: Sit up close enough to the end of the tub so that your feet are braced. Your legs are fully extended. Stretch the arms out parallel in front of you, with fingers close together and palms facing.
  1. Pull in your abdominals, elongate the back, and reach forward. Back upright, look ahead.
  2. Relax for a few seconds and sit back.
  3. Continue reaching forward, a bit further each time in a bouncing motion. Careful—though it is easier to stretch in warm water, do it with tender loving care.

Helpful Hints: Imagine that you are the puppet again with the strings attached to the tips of your fingers—and those strings were pulling you forward!
  Make sure you relax properly between stretches.

Après
Shower and Bath

Having stepped out of your shower or bath and dried yourself thoroughly (a bit of talc perhaps to absorb excess body moisture or after-bath lotion for extra skin care), you're ready to complete your daily stretches. Here's where you are in for a pleasant surprise! Now that you've loosened up a bit, increased the blood circulation, and let go of a lot of undue muscle tension, you will find yourself easing into the exercises almost naturally. And you'll be ready to limber up for the day's activities without moaning and groaning from early morning stiffness.

Here are nine basic towel stretches. Once you've learned them, you will find you can run through them within a few minutes.

Since you've taken the time to warm those muscles you certainly won't want to let them cool off. So slip into something warm, comfortable, *and* practical that will cover the arms and legs. I personally use a two-piece terry warm-up suit—it's ideal—but a leotard and tights, or loose-fitting slacks and a warm shirt will do just as well for you to exercise in.

I hope you will be able to remain in the warm bathroom. But since you'll need enough space to lie out on the floor, or swing your arms and legs while standing, the bedroom may prove more suitable for you. Any carpeted area or rug is fine for these exercises, but please, don't do your stretches on a cold floor!

For the towel series you will need to have a towel handy. (A bath-size towel is fine for most of the exercises. You can adjust your grip on the towel to suit your needs.)

Take your time—practice an exercise a few times before going on to the next. Check alignment before each exercise to allow muscles to work harmoniously —in that way you will insure stability. And make these exercises a daily routine so that you'll maintain the flexibility you have worked so hard to achieve.

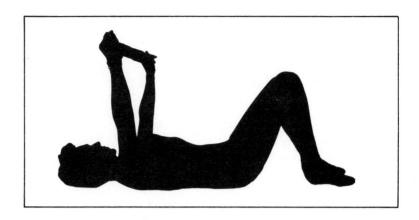

Pelvic Tilt—Rib Cage Lift

For: Flexibility of the pelvis; aligning the spine; strengthening the derrière and abdominals; stretching the arms and upper back

Here's where we combine the Supine Pelvic Tilt with an upper torso stretch—the Pelvic Tilt will always be my number-one exercise. Doing it from the supine position is *the* best way to practice it; here it's combined with a towel stretch to work the muscles in the arms, shoulders, and upper back as well. As your arms should be as far apart as possible, you'll need a large towel for this one.

Preparation: Lie in a supine position on the floor. Knees are bent and feet parallel and shoulder-width apart. Remember to tuck the chin in slightly. Clasp a towel in both hands, holding it firmly at either end, until the towel is taut when you place it across your chest.

1. Pinch the derrière together as you tighten the abdominals and tilt your pelvis, holding the contraction. At the same time raise the towel straight up above your head, then over the head until the towel rests on the floor behind you.

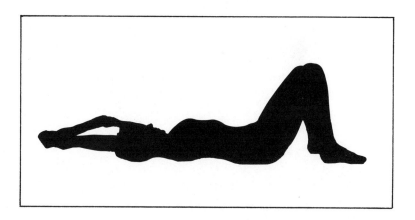

2. Bend the elbows and bring the towel forward again to the neutral position; as you do so, release the contraction, relax, and let go.

3. Repeat these two movements at least five times, bringing the towel up and over your head as you tilt the pelvis, then bringing it back across your chest as you relax the pelvis onto the floor.

After you have repeated this exercise and feel comfortable doing it, add the Rib Cage Lift.

4. Clasp the towel and place it across the chest.

5. Now breathe in slowly and deeply, bringing the towel up and over your head; then B-L-O-W out just as slowly as you bring it back again.

6. Repeat the exercise several times, doing first the Pelvic Tilt, then the Rib Cage Lift with rhythmic breathing.

Helpful Hint: The deeper you breathe in, the more the exercise works into the rib cage; and the more air you blow out, the deeper you are reaching those lower back muscles, flattening the back into the floor. It also gives you a good stretch in the shoulder and upper back muscles.

Body Roll (1)

For: Aligning, stretching, and strengthening the spine

This exercise is the ultimate for back flexibility, for it stretches the entire spine, vertebra by vertebra. Prepare by first doing your shower and bath exercises, then supine pelvic tilt and leg stretch to make sure your back muscles are loose. Imagine yourself moving like a rocking chair here, as it starts slowly and gradually picks up momentum. The towel will brace your arms and keep the body well-centered and balanced. Naturally the more you relax, the easier you'll find this.

Preparation: Sit on the floor with your knees bent and your feet shoulder-distance apart. Place the towel under your knees, and palms facing toward you, grasp it firmly at either end. Look down at the floor.

1. Breathe in to prepare. Tucking your chin in slightly, pull the towel up and lift your feet off the floor.

2. B-L-O-W out slowly, and at the same time, lean back pulling at the towel as you roll back onto the floor. Keep the arms in close to your body and remain in a fetal position. Don't try going back too far the first few times. It is better to warm up a bit first.

3. Breathe in slowly then exhale as you roll forward and return to the seated position.

4. B-L-O-W out again, tugging at the towel a bit harder and letting yourself roll back far enough so that your knees are just over your head.

5. Breathe in and roll back as before.

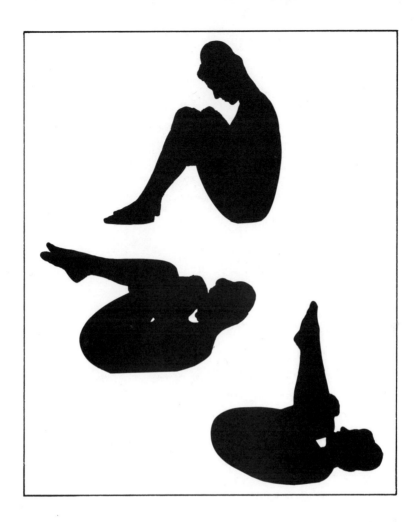

6. Repeat these two movements, feeling yourself rocking back and forth until you're loose enough to let the knees drop right over your head and your toes touch the floor.

Helpful Hint: Gravity and momentum work well here. As the weight of your legs roll you back, you stretch your upper back muscles; as the weight of your head and shoulders rolls you forward, you are stretching the lower back muscles. Combine this with a towel and rhythmic breathing—and it's not difficult at all!

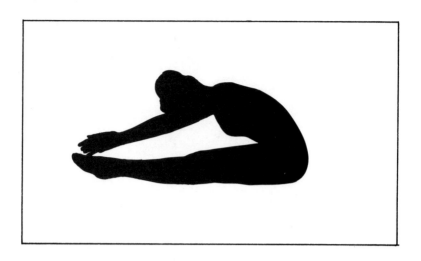

Body Roll (2)

For: Aligning, stretching, and strengthening the spine

This is a variation of the previous exercise, with the addition of a thigh stretch. This time you won't need a towel. Repeat the first Body Roll until you're comfortable with it, then you will be ready for this one.

Preparation: Sit on the floor with knees bent and clasp your knees with your hands. Breathe in gently.

1. Breathe out slowly and at the same time roll back as far as possible.

2. Breathe in, then out as you roll up again. When your feet touch the floor, slide them forward and let your arms and torso follow.

3. Clasp your knees again, breathe in to prepare, then out as you roll back.

4. Roll up again. Keep the arms parallel and palms facing each other as you let the weight of your head and shoulders pull your body down toward the legs.

5. Relax and repeat the entire exercise.

6. If you really feel you can do this with ease, then

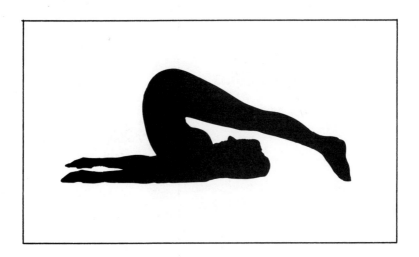

you are ready to do a more extensive body stretch. From sitting position, with legs fully extended, this time breathe in slowly; as you B-L-O-W out, roll back lifting the legs up and over, keeping them straight and together. Don't be afraid of letting them touch the floor in back of you, before you roll up once more as in step 4. Relax completely before repeating again.

Helpful Hint: You can repeat this Body Roll several times if you feel like it. But keep the rocking movement continuous; don't hold either the forward or back position. And remember to breathe out as you roll back and again, as you roll up.

Here I have chosen some special exercises that can effectively be practiced using your towel rack, the edge of a wash basin, dressing table, or any counter surface that will provide adequate support. I prefer the towel rack because it gives you good leverage. But whatever you choose, double-check before using it; make sure that it is secure.

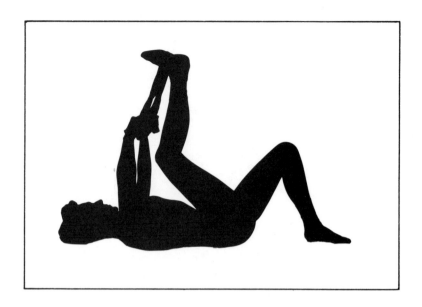

Leg Stretch

For: Stretching the hamstring muscles

Since the hamstrings begin at the pelvis and continue down the back of the thighs, their elasticity affects the flexibility of the lower back muscles. Exercises stretching the hamstrings are the ones we tend to dislike the most because hamstrings are normally tight and a bit painful to stretch. You'll find that after the bath hamstrings will stretch with greater ease and less discomfort. A towel to brace the arms is a big help.

Preparation: Sit up on the floor with the knees bent. Take a towel and place it under the instep of your right foot, grasping it on either side close to your ankle.

1. Roll onto your back, keeping the left leg on the floor, and bend your right knee in toward the chest, still holding the towel firmly with both hands.

2. Keeping the right foot flexed, slowly and gently

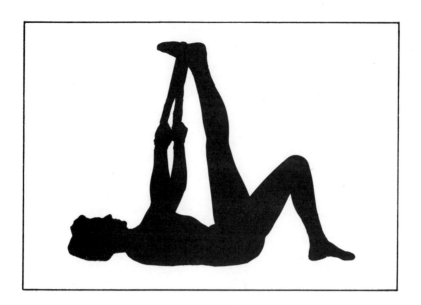

straighten the knee upward and pull the leg toward you in a slow rocking motion.

3. Continue pulling the leg toward you, gently but firmly.

4. Still grasping the towel, bend your elbows and bring the knee in to your chest again, then push the foot up toward the ceiling, trying to straighten the knee as much as you can.

5. Continue bending and straightening the leg a few more times.

6. Repeat these two stretches several times—pulling the leg forward and back, then bending and stretching it up, using the towel as a sling.

7. Put the right leg down; repeat the exercise with the left leg.

Helpful Hints: As you rock the leg, try to let go of any tightness in the neck and shoulders (closing the eyes often helps). The more you can relax, the better the stretch.

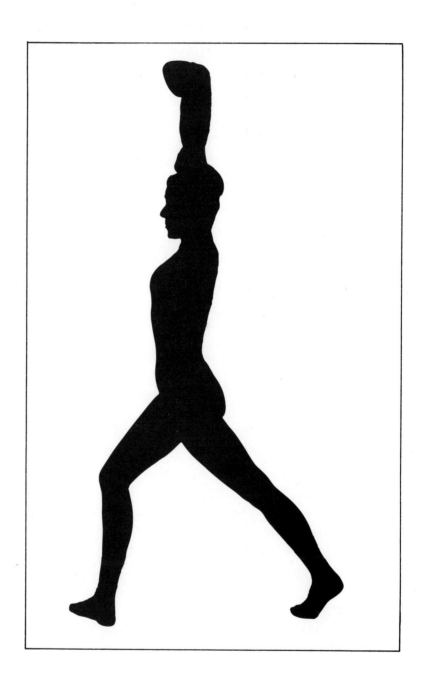

Forward Lunge

For: Stretching the thighs and Achilles tendon; stretching the arms and upper torso

Here's a dual-purpose exercise for thighs *and* the Achilles tendon, where stretching and conditioning is essential, especially for active sports. An ounce of prevention is worth a pound of cure, and this is good for preventing muscle injuries. High-heeled shoes can shorten Achilles tendons, so if you wear them, these exercises are a must!

Preparation: Stand tall and grasp the towel firmly in both hands. Raise your arms stretching them over your head as far apart as possible.

1. In one movement, bend the right leg and lunge forward onto the right foot with toes turned out a little, taking as large a step as you comfortably can. Keep the knee bent but the torso erect.

2. Keeping the arms raised high, shift your weight back a little.

3. Now lunge forward even farther, aiming for a deeper bend (it's like a fencer's pose), without bending the torso. The deeper the knee bend, the greater the stretch to the thigh and the Achilles tendon.

4. Repeat this lunge eight or ten times. Relax, bring feet together, and rest a few seconds.

5. Alternate feet and lunge with the left foot.

Helpful Hint: It's important to think of elongation and keep the back well aligned.

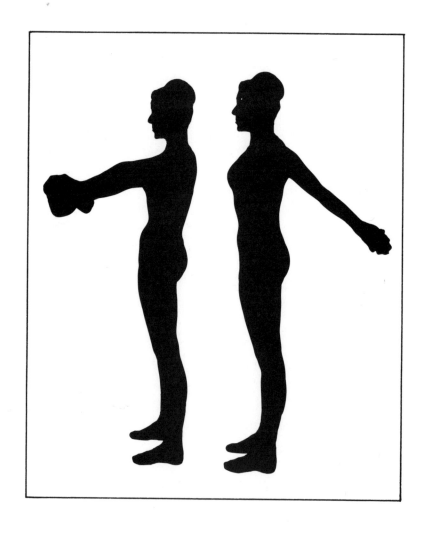

Roll Over

For: Stretching the upper back and shoulders; firming the bosom

Even if you've always had good posture, this

stretch will help you maintain flexibility in the shoulders and upper back, so essential for tennis, golf, or almost any active sport.

Preparation: Grasp a large bath towel firmly at both ends and hold it out in front of you at waist level. Relax the head and neck.

1. Breathe in, and as you do so, lift the towel straight up above your head.

2. Breathe out, and bending the elbows slightly, stretch the towel behind you and down to thigh level.

3. Breathe in again and pull the towel up over the head.

4. Breathe out again to pull the towel forward to its original position.

5. Repeat at least three times. Try to do this without bending the elbows more than is necessary to get the towel over the head.

Helpful Hints: Aim for keeping your arms as straight as you can, but avoid any strain. Keep the derrière as tight as possible—it helps to prevent your back from overarching and reduces possible strain.

If you can do this exercise with the elbows straight, then you are limber enough to shorten the grip on the towel by bringing your hands closer together.

When doing an exercise that takes as much effort as this one can, you may inadvertently tighten the muscles in the neck and shoulders. Try to check this from time to time by doing a few Head Rotations to loosen the neck muscles.

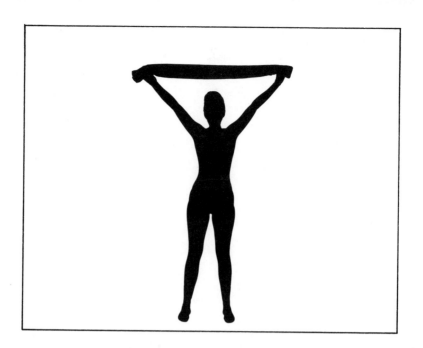

Side Bend Stretch

For: Stretching the sides of the torso; slimming the waist; stretching the arms and upper back

The trick to bending is to relax and let gravity pull you down. When you include rhythmic breathing too, you've got everything going for you. It's good to breathe in before starting, then bend as you breathe out. Here's a thought to hold on to whenever you combine breathing and bending: Breathe in to prepare, breathe out till you're there!

Preparation: Stand up and check to make sure your feet are parallel and shoulder-distance apart. Grasping the towel at each end, raise it directly above your head. Keep the arms straight and relax your head and neck.

1. Breathe in slowly; as you B-L-O-W out, pull the towel down with your right hand as your shoulder

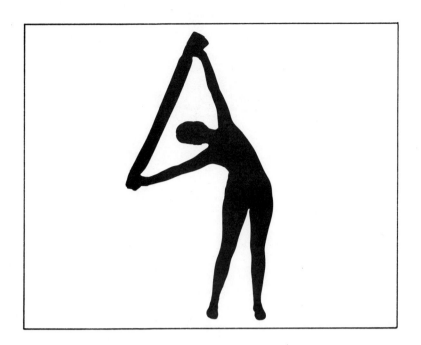

drops down and your head tilts to the right. Try not to resist, but relax and let go as you bend your torso.

2. B-L-O-W in again, and with your left hand pulling the towel this time, lift your head and torso to the neutral position, arms outstretched overhead.

3. Breathe out as slowly as possible, and with the left hand leading, repeat the bend to the left side.

4. Repeat both side bends three more times.

Helpful Hints: Try to keep your head and shoulders in line with your hips, bending to each side in one piece, without twisting the torso. Remember the metronome as you move rhythmically and fluidly in one plane. While you are in the side bend you can get an extra little stretch by giving an added pull on the towel to get you down a bit farther. You can do this side stretch anywhere, with or without a towel. Try it sitting in an armless chair with your arms hanging loosely down at your sides; as you bend from side to side feel your fingers reaching down for the floor.

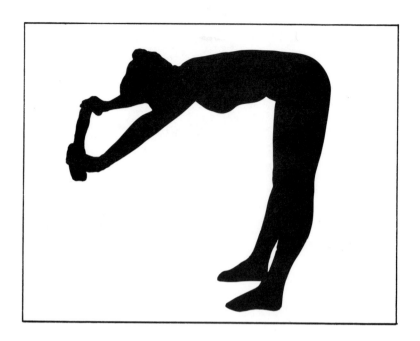

Bend Over—Roll Up

For: Slimming the waist; stretching the thighs and lower back; aligning the spine

This is both a stretching and a relaxing exercise. It's a little strenuous but well worth the effort. The towel helps you maintain full extension of the upper back and that's what gives you a good stretch.

Preparation: Check your alignment and pull in those abdominals so that you are standing firmly and well-balanced. Feet are parallel, with toes pointing forward. Grasp the towel at each end and hold it up above the head, arms outstretched.

1. Breathe in slowly; then as you begin to B-L-O-W out, bend forward from the hips keeping your arms above your head. Looking down at the floor, continue bending until you have gone as far down as you can with your legs still straight.

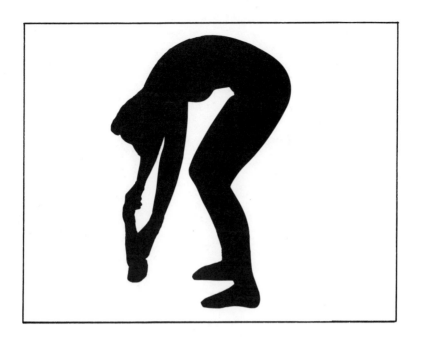

2. Bend your knees and relax your arms, letting the towel drop down. As you begin to breathe in again, roll up slowly, pressing your feet into the floor, pulling in the abdominals, and relaxing the shoulders. Come up one section at a time—lower back, middle back, and finally the upper back—as you do the Roll Up stretch, lifting the head up last as you raise the towel over the head again.

3. Repeat the whole movement, bending from the hips as you go down, rolling up from the hips as you come up. Try to remain very relaxed and you'll feel yourself doing it in one continuous undulating motion.

Helpful Hint: As you become familiar with this exercise, you'll discover how well the movement flows with rhythmic breathing—a good example of the compatibility of effort and action.

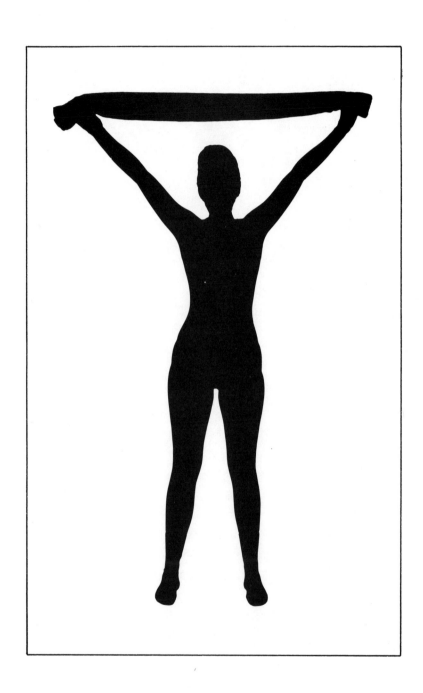

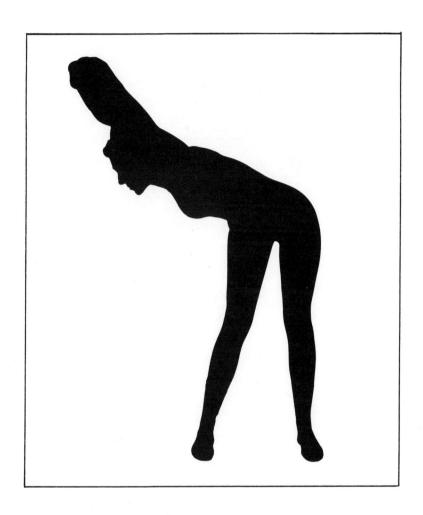

The Big O

For: Stretching the back; flexibility of the torso; slimming the waist

Here's another fine example of how the upper back moves independently from the lower back, as

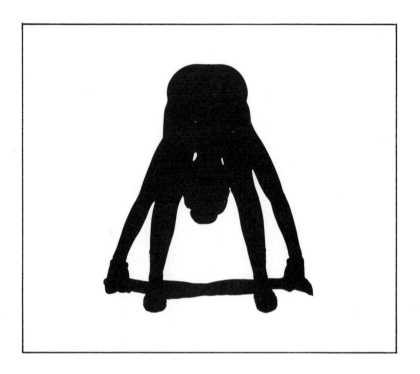

parts of a puppet will. The head, arms, and upper back move as one piece (yes, it will take a little concentration and control) while the lower torso remains still. By doing this we get an even greater stretch, especially in that hard-to-reach waist area. This is a wonderful warm-up for any active sport, especially golf and tennis.

Preparation: Stand up, in alignment, with your knees straight. Grasping a towel firmly, hold it over your head. The arms remain stretched throughout this exercise.

1. Breathe in slowly and twist the upper body to the right.

2. B-L-O-W out and drop your torso down, pulling the towel forward and down just outside the right leg.

3. Swing the towel, keeping it parallel to the floor, across in front of your feet to the left side. Try not to bend the knees here.

4. Breathe in again, and tighten the derrière and abdominals. Continue breathing in as you pull up the towel to an overhead position and turn to face forward.

5. Repeat the whole exercise, this time reversing sides. Begin by twisting the body to the left, then swing down and through, coming up on the right side.

6. Repeat the swing several more times on each side. B-L-O-W out as you bend down, breathe in as you lift up.

Helpful Hints: When you stand up, make sure your hips and legs are centered over your feet and that your feet feel as if they were glued to the floor! It really helps.

The towel describes a circle, so aim to make it a big O! Holding the towel up over your head makes a difference because the torso *lifts up* before it *bends over* to get the maximum stretch. Keep the movement fluid, while you relax and enjoy it.

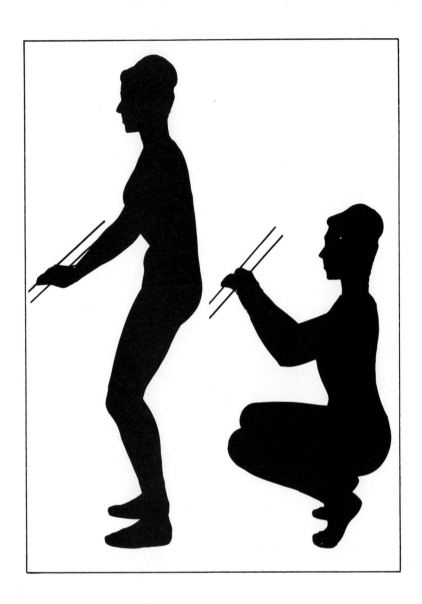

Knee Bends

For: Leg flexibility

Knees are vulnerable to injury. Since so many people today participate in active sports, it's well worth the effort to do at least one exercise that will keep the knees conditioned. This one is dual purpose in that it tones up the thighs too. You'll find that the shower and bath exercises prepare you well for this one!

Preparation: Stand with feet slightly apart and hold on to the towel rack or sink.

1. Tighten the derrière muscles, pull in the navel, and at the same time begin to bend the knees.

2. Continue to bend, going down as far as you can without lifting your heels off the floor. You'll feel as though the derrière muscles are pulling the legs down. Make sure the back remains erect and shoulders don't droop forward.

3. Come up slowly, but as you do *resist* straightening the legs by pressing your heels into the floor as you pull the knees in. When you get to the point where the legs are straight again, rest and relax a few seconds, then repeat once more.

4. Begin to bend the knees once more as in Step 2. As you tighten your abdominals, go down as far as you can with heels still on the floor, then lift the heels and continue going down farther. Make sure your back is elongated during the entire exercise.

5. As you slowly come back up you can use your abdominals to help get you there, thus putting less strain on your knees.

Helpful Hint: Pinch—Pull really works when you are using resistance to get those thigh muscles working —and that's what makes this exercise so effective.

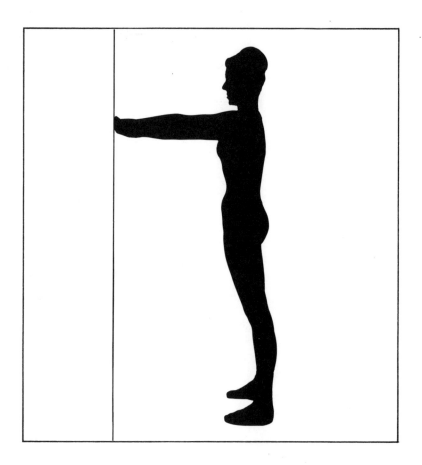

Push Away

For: Strengthening the upper arms, stretching the Achilles tendon

This upper arm stretch not only firms the arms to prevent flabbiness, but strengthens those muscles and prepares them for active sports. Use the bathroom door or any wall for firm support and good leverage.

Preparation: With feet together, stand an arm's length away from the wall. Place hands against wall and spread them apart, turning the thumbs in toward one another.

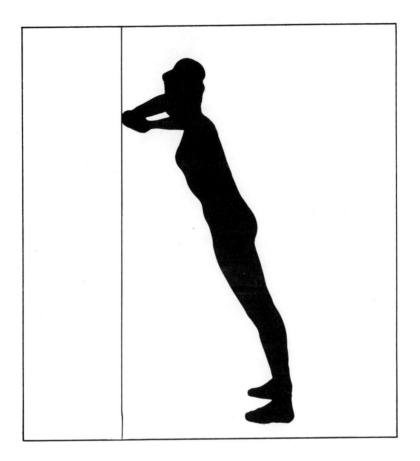

1. Bend the elbows and let your torso fall forward, keeping back and legs straight.

2. Continue bending until the elbows point directly to each side.

3. Push against the wall with your hands as you push up and back with the torso.

4. Repeat this motion of falling forward-pushing back several times.

Helpful Hints: For a deeper stretch, include a breathing pattern here: Breathe in to prepare; breathe out as you drop forward, then breathe in again as you push back.

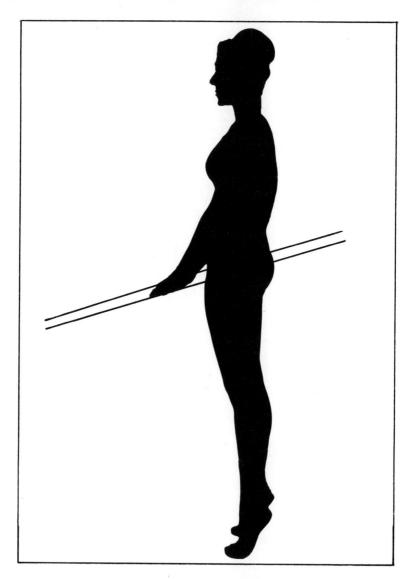

Foot Rolls

For: Strengthening muscles in the foot and lower leg; strengthening the derrière and abdominals '

Here's one that not only strengthens the muscles in the feet—which we tend to neglect and sometimes abuse—but also tightens the calves.

Preparation: Hold on to a towel rack or wash basin.

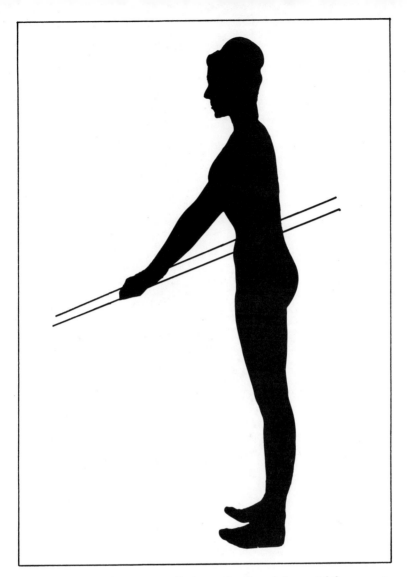

Stand with feet parallel and shoulder-width apart, with your weight centered over the instep. Tighten your derrière and abdominals.

1. Roll up onto the balls of your feet, keeping the knees as straight as possible.

2. Roll down and back onto your heels, raising the toes so that they come up off the floor.

3. Repeat these two movements—rolling forward and up, rolling down and back—at least eight times.

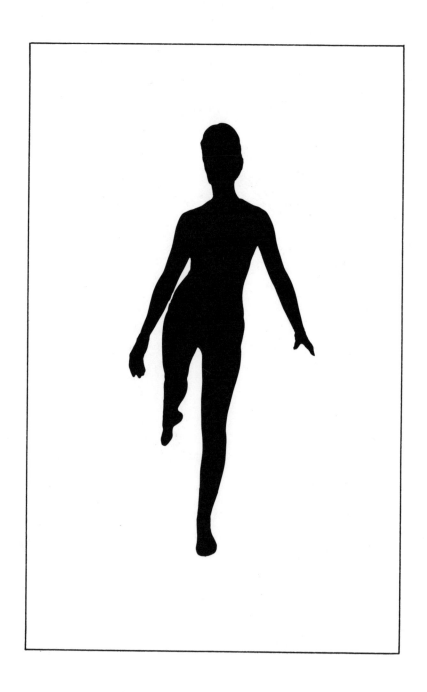

Leg Swings

For: Tightening thighs; strengthening the lower back; tightening the derrière muscles

The focus of this exercise is not on how *high* the leg lifts up, but on how controlled the swing is. And keep control by using pinch-pull.

Preparation: Turn sideways and hold on to the rack or sink with the left hand. Stand in good alignment, tightening the derrière, pulling in the navel, with your weight on the left leg. The right arm hangs loosely down at the side.

1. Swing the right leg forward and up.

2. Bring it down to just off the floor and swing it back as far as it will go without bending the knee. Keep the body straight to avoid arching the back.

3. Continue this pendulum swing eight to ten times, swinging the leg as freely as possible as it goes forward and back. As the foot drops down it will feel as though it's sweeping the floor. It's a continuous, very fluid motion.

4. Turn to face the opposite direction, holding on to the rack with the right hand. Repeat the swing with the other leg.

Helpful Hint: Look straight ahead and remember to elongate the back.

Special Exercises for Special Needs

Now it's time for a few exercises for special areas that always seem to need attention, to suit your particular needs. Look through them all and decide which ones will benefit you most. They can be done at virtually any time, so keep them on hand for whenever you need them.

The isometrics work like a charm and travel well too. The exercises for hands and feet are a blessing for stiff joints (many women are *naturally* tight in their joints); I would suggest that you check with your doctor before doing them if you have any doubts about whether they are suitable for you. The "on-the-spot" relaxers are beneficial for everyone and suitable for any time of day.

If it's possible for you to do some of the standing exercises in front of a mirror, take advantage of it. The mirror will help you understand what your body is doing and I can't think of a better way to remind you about posture. Once you see how easy it is to align, you can become your own teacher as you observe and correct!

Here's a last-minute reminder. All the exercises are really as easy as ABC—and that means

> Align your body
> Breathe slowly and fluidly
> Concentrate but relax!

Please don't neglect the exercises because you are too busy or not in the mood. That may be just the time when you need them most.

I am particularly fond of these first two stretches because they work well together for limbering up the shoulders and arms. If I were going to play tennis or golf, or any other sport for that matter, I wouldn't leave home without doing them. If you grasp a washcloth in either hand as you do them, you'll also be toning and strengthening the arms.

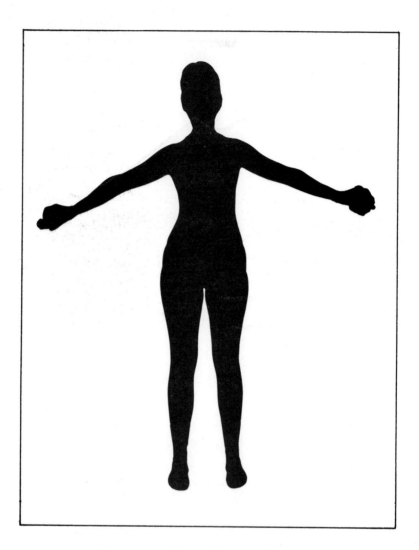

▬▬ Over the Rainbow ⌄

For: Stretching the shoulders and upper back

This works best when you include a breathing pattern. Try it when you first get out of bed in the morning—it's delicious!

Preparation: Stand up in good alignment grasping a washcloth in each hand (this is optional, not essential). Arms are stretched out to the sides, palms upward.

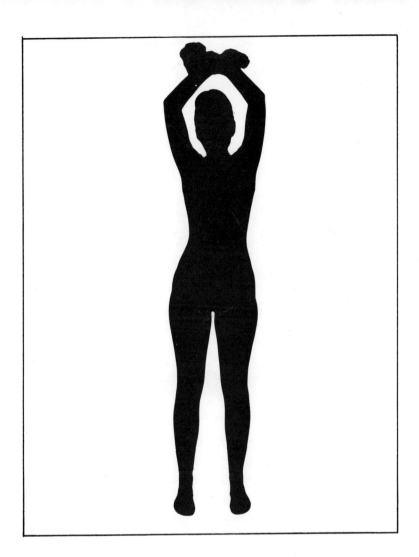

1. Breathe in slowly and lift the arms up over your head until hands cross each other.

2. Now turn the hands away from each other; as you B-L-O-W out, slowly press the arms down to the sides.

3. Repeat these two movements—pulling up and pressing down—three more times, describing a large semicircle with each arm.

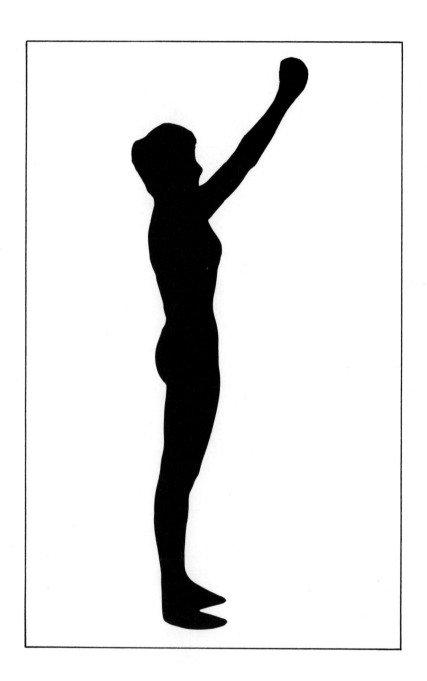

The Backstroke

For: Stretching the upper back

Preparation: Stand up in good alignment, arms down by your sides, grasping a washcloth in each hand (again, the washcloth is optional), palms facing up.

1. Breathe in, and as you do, swing the right arm forward and up until it's extended above the head.
2. Turn the hand so that the palm faces back; as you B-L-O-W out, reach the arm back then pull it down to your side again.
3. Repeat the action with the left arm.
4. Repeat at least once more with both arms.

Helpful Hint: For a maximum stretch, keep facing forward, isolating the movement so that the head doesn't turn with the shoulders.

Side-to-Side Pull

For: Stretching the upper arms and shoulders

Here's an exercise for the upper arms and shoulders that is a bit strenuous, but terrific! You use a washcloth here for resistance, so the muscles get a good workout. If you have sufficient room, do it while you're in the shower and take advantage of the warm water spray; if not, try it as soon as you have finished bathing.

Preparation: Grasp a washcloth at either end; lift it up over your head, bending your elbows, and place the cloth directly behind your head. Tuck the chin in and try to keep your neck relaxed throughout.

1. Grasp the cloth firmly with your left hand as your right hand pulls the cloth down toward the right shoulder.

2. Relax your grasp a bit; now pull down with your left hand over the left shoulder.

3. Repeat several times, pulling from right to left.

Helpful Hint: Don't overdo the pulling here—it's quite a stretch!

Here's a multipurpose exercise that focuses on the legs and feet. Our knees and the thigh muscles that protect them are very vulnerable—and this exercise is ideal for toning up the thighs. Warm-ups for the legs and feet are essential prior to active sports, especially

118

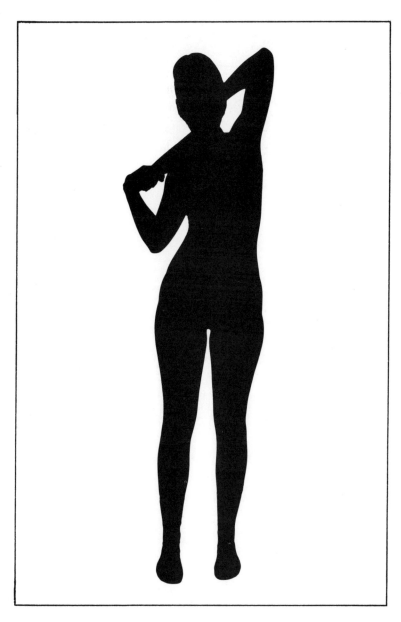

when the weather turns damp and cold. So here's the chance to strengthen muscles that you depend on but often neglect. It's also a good reminder of how important it is to have strong abdominals.

Pedal Push

For: Stretching and strengthening the thighs, ankles, and toes

Where: Sitting or standing

Preparation: Sit up in a chair, as far back as possible to give your back good support, or use the toilet seat in the bathroom to sit on. Brace hands on seat.

1. Stretch the right leg out in front of you until the knee straightens.

2. Flex the right foot by pulling it in toward you as far as possible (toes will now point directly upward).

3. Now raise the right leg just enough so that it is no longer touching the seat. Here's the time to concentrate on pinch-pull!

4. Stretch the toes forward and rotate the foot, circling twice to the right, then twice to the left.

5. Flex the foot again. Pull in the navel to get the abdominals working, and as you do so, bend the knee slowly in toward you, bringing it as close to your body as possible.

6. Relax and drop the leg to its original position. Repeat with the left leg.

7. Repeat at least twice more with each leg.

Helpful Hint: When you are in a car or airplane and can't find room to fully extend your legs, try the flex,

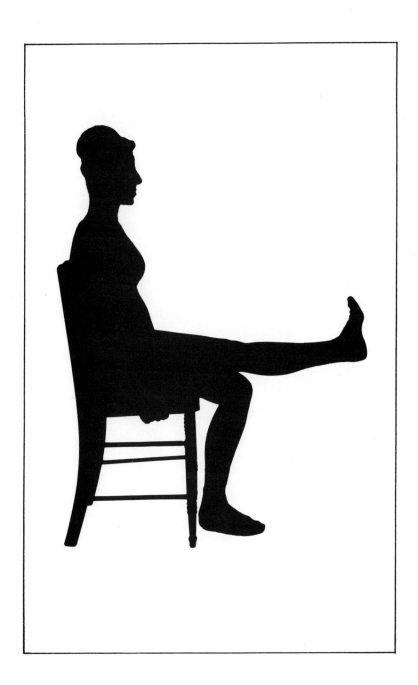

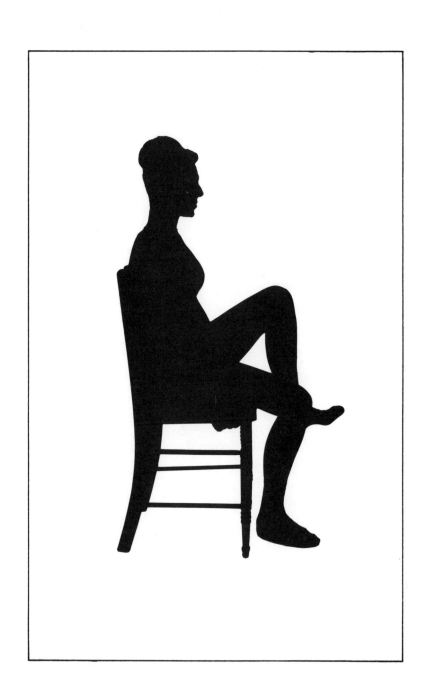

stretch, and rotation of the foot—it's a great traveling companion for long trips!

Few people escape the usual problems related to the aging process. One of the most common is stiffening of the joints, particularly in cold, damp climates. But keeping those joints loose and limber improves mobility and helps reduce the calcium deposits that form. I have a bit of arthritis myself and can appreciate what gentle exercising will do.

Our extremities seem to suffer the most. Yet what do we do for our neglected hands and feet? One answer is to take advantage of the pulsating spray from the shower and do some hand exercises. And the bath is ideal, too, for exercising feet under running water. In both cases, increasing the circulation to the muscles helps considerably. So I'm including here the exercises I have found to be best.

Hand Stretches

1. This is a great one. Hold a large sponge (at least one and one half inches thick) in one hand, squeeze it hard together, then release the squeeze to relax the hand. Repeat at least ten times—and remember it's the *release* that's important.

2. As if you were playing castanets, bend down one finger at a time—start with the little finger and end with the thumb—toward the palm of your hand, then straighten your fingers and begin again. Continue bending and straightening one finger after another, in one fluid movement.

3. Bend your elbows and put your hands together in front of your chest, fingers and thumbs touching only (as if you were praying). Without letting the palms touch, press the fingers in toward each other, then release. Continue this pressing together a few times—imagine that you had a small ball between your hands that you were squeezing.

4. Alternating with each hand, describe large circles with your wrist, first in a clockwise direction, then counterclockwise.

5. Grasp each finger of the right hand, one at a time, with the left hand, and pull gently. Repeat with the left hand.

▬ The Gripper ▼

This foot exercise is really excellent. I'd suggest you do it standing on the floor or seated in the bathroom. Place a wash cloth on the floor.

1. With your right foot, grip and hold on to a washcloth with your toes, raising it just off the floor.

2. Hold for a few seconds then release it.

3. Relax and repeat gripping and releasing with the left foot.

4. Repeat this a few more times.

The following two exercises are wonderful to do while you are relaxing in the bath.

▬ Flex and Stretch ▼

Preparation: Sit up tall in the bath with legs outstretched. Hold on to the side of the tub for support; relax head and shoulders and focus on your foot movement.

1. Flex the right foot, toes pointing straight up to the ceiling. The more you pull the foot toward you, the greater the stretch.

2. Now point the toes as you press them down.

3. Continue flexing and pointing the foot; it will describe an arc as it moves back and forth.

4. Repeat a few times, then relax and repeat with the left foot.

▬ Foot Circles ⌄

This is very good for maintaining flexibility in the ankles, especially when it's cold. It is a good exercise to do before any sport that involves running.

Preparation: Sit in the tub with legs extended, knees slightly bent. Focus now on the big toe of your right foot.

1. Rotate the right foot in a clockwise circle, making as large a circle as possible.
2. Rotate it four times, then relax.
3. Repeat these rotations with the left foot.

The following are *isometrics*, exercises that produce deep contractions of the muscles without involving any movement. Since isometrics will build muscle tension for you (and in fact are supposed to do that), I can't stress strongly enough how essential it is to concentrate on the letting-go action, releasing the tension after each exercise.

Because they do so much for toning muscles that keep the body in shape, isometrics are good to know. These two isometrics are among my favorites, and will really hit the spot!

(Isometrics may be harmful to anyone with a heart problem, so please check with your doctor before doing these exercises if you have any reason to suspect that you should eliminate them.

▬ Hand Press ▼

For: Toning the pectoral muscles; firming the breast and upper arms

This is a gem and can be done anywhere. Do it in the shower or do it in the tub, but do it every day. If you want to see for yourself how the muscles respond, try it for the first time in front of your mirror, *without* clothes of course.

Preparation: Sitting in the tub, or standing in the shower, bend your arms and place your hands directly in front of your chest, with the left palm facing you and the right palm facing away.

1. Now place the butt of one hand (the area just under the thumb) across the other, hands still apart.

2. Press the butts against each other as firmly as you can as though you were crushing a nut between them. Hold for a count of six. Release, relax and let go.

3. Reverse the position of your hands, the left palm facing away and the right palm facing toward you this time.

4. Repeat the pressing-together action.

5. Repeat again, reversing hand directions once more.

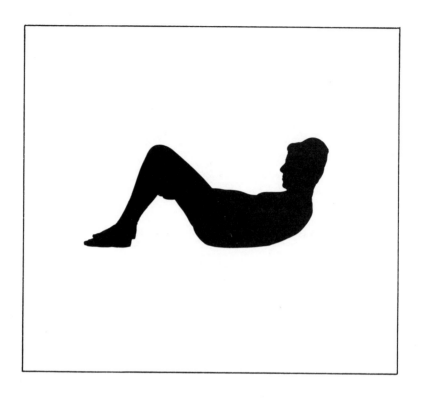

Mini-Sit-Up

For: Strengthening the abdominals; flattening the tummy

I'm sure you are all familiar with sit-ups. Here I'm giving them to you as a "mini" exercise; I think these are better than the regular sit-ups because you will be lifting just one third of the way, far enough so that the abdominals do all the work, but not so far that the back muscles begin to take over! You'll find this exercise extremely effective. Although it is only partially an isometric, it is a really powerful one. It is particularly good for the woman who can't feel the abdominals working when she's doing the Dynamic Exercise. The contraction helps build tone faster.

Preparation: Lie on the floor, with knees bent and feet parallel and shoulder-distance apart. Place your arms at your sides, palms toward the body. Breathe in and out slowly, relaxing completely.

1. Breathe in again as slowly as possible.

2. As you begin to B-L-O-W out, drop the head forward (tucking in the chin). As if someone were pulling your hands forward, begin to roll up as you lift your arms, shoulders, and upper back off the floor (about where your bra strap would be).

3. Without moving any part of the body, hold that position for at least six seconds and breathe normally. I think you've got the message by now!

4. Roll back down and rest for a few seconds.

5. Repeat this exercise several more times, trying to hold the contraction a few seconds longer — and try to keep any tension from creeping into the neck by consciously relaxing.

Helpful Hint: You may feel your muscles quiver — that's OK. Once you've built up tone, your muscles won't have to work so hard.

The following two are isotonics, rather than isometrics; they involve contraction of the muscles with some movement involved.

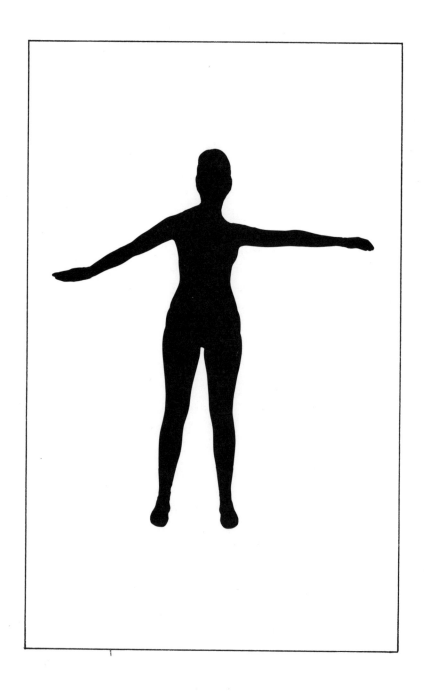

▬ Arm Twist ⌐

This is an exercise for tightening that little flabbiness in the upper arm. It also works into the shoulders and upper back.

1. Stand up; stretch your arms out to the sides, palms up. With the little finger leading, turn the right hand under until the palm faces up again, rotating the shoulder. At the same time press the shoulder down as firmly as possible until you can feel the muscles tighten.

2. With the thumb leading, untwist the hand and return to first position, pressing down with the shoulder again.

3. Repeat this four times, rotating the arms and pressing down with the shoulder.

4. Repeat again with the left arm.

Chin Chopper

The flabbiness right below the chin is more prevalent in some women than in others. If you have a suspicion of sag, here's an exercise to help. It's beneficial to do this one several times a day, in front of the mirror as you brush your teeth or even in the bath or shower.

1. Sit up tall and lift your head toward the ceiling.
2. Open your mouth and push the jaws forward.
3. Without closing the lips, begin a chewing motion with the jaws.
4. Repeat several times until you feel the muscles tightening under your chin.
5. Relax completely.

Here are some nice stretches that are good for early in the morning as you're getting up, or if you're confined to bed for a time. A good night's sleep is a blessing, but lying in any one position all night can cause the muscles to tighten and cramp. Let these few exercises "unlock" that cramped feeling. Notice how even a dog or cat will stretch its limbs after it has been sleeping for a long time!

Other excellent exercises to practice in bed are the Knee and Ankle Hug, the pelvic tilt and The Slapper.

If you can't fit a shower or bath into your daily routine, but do want to prepare for the towel exercises, these are a must!

⬛ Neck Roll ⌄

For: Loosening the neck muscles

Where: In bed

Preparation: Remove the pillow and lie flat on your back, with knees bent and arms by your sides.

1. Tuck your chin in and roll your head slowly to the right. As you turn, your chin should be reaching for the right shoulder.

2. Keeping the chin tucked in, roll the head back to the center over toward the left shoulder. It will be drawing an arc as your head drops and swivels around.

3. Repeat three times, moving the head slowly and fluidly.

Helpful Hint: Each time you tuck in your chin (without tightening the neck muscles) you can be sure that your head is in good alignment. So whenever you feel a crick in your neck, try this to relieve it.

The Neck Stretch is also good when done seated in a chair; close your eyes to help relax tension.

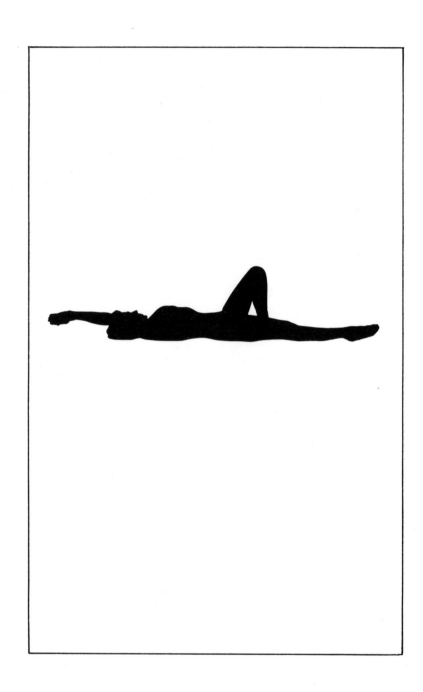

Supine Body Stretch

For: Stretching the torso

Where: In bed or lying on the floor (the bed you use must have a firm mattress or the exercise will not be as beneficial)

This one is especially effective as an early morning stretch. Or repeat it anytime lying on the floor, especially after you've warmed your back muscles in the shower.

Preparation: Remove the pillow and slide down far enough so that you can extend an arm over your head (if you still don't have enough room, try this on the diagonal). Bend the left leg, but keep the right one extended. The left arm is at your side, the right one directly behind your head.

1. Imagine that strings were tied around both wrists and that someone was pulling both of them at the same time in opposite directions. Pull your right arm back (even farther) as you pull the left arm forward—and feel the stretch from stem to stern.

2. Relax a second and repeat twice more.

3. Reverse the position of arms and legs, and repeat to the left side.

Hip Roll

For: Loosening the lower back muscles

Where: In bed or lying on the floor

There's no better way to keep the lower back limber than by stretching it independently from the upper back. The bed is an ideal place to do this, since you can grasp on to the edge of the mattress and stabilize the upper torso, isolating the movement. If you want to repeat the exercise on the floor, you will be firming the hips, arms, and bosom as well.

Preparation: Lie on your back and bring the knees up to the chest, toes pointed down. If you're on a single bed, grasp the sides of the mattress with both hands as resistance. If the bed's too wide, grasp with one hand only.

1. Roll the knees over to the right, and at the same time, turn your head to the left.

2. Relax and bring them forward again.

3. Repeat to the other side, knees to the left, head to the right.

4. Continue rolling from side to side, with head and knees moving in opposition.

Helpful Hints: Remember to keep the knees together and shoulders flat on the bed.

Try this exercise with a breathing pattern: Breathe in when the head and knees are facing forward, and B-L-O-W out when they roll to the sides.

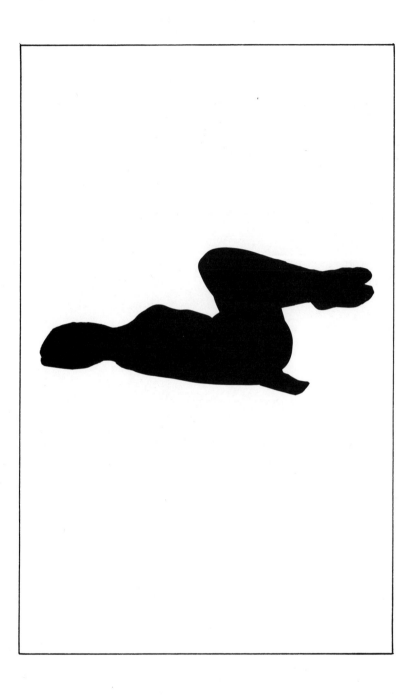

▬ Shoulder Stretch ⌄

For: Loosening the upper back muscles

Where: Sitting on the bed, or anywhere

Here's a way to work out shoulder cramps or upper back tightness. Since this is so worthwhile, repeat it whenever you get that tired, achy feeling in your upper back. It's similar to the Shoulder Rotations (Chapter 2) except that here you get a deeper stretch.

Preparation: Sit on the edge of the bed with your hands in your lap. Relax the head and neck. Shrug your shoulders a few times to relax tension.

1. Imagine that your right shoulder was trying to touch (a) the wall in front of you, (b) the ceiling, (c) the wall right behind you, and (d) the floor. Now quite slowly, press your shoulder forward, lift it up, pull it back, and drop it down—holding each movement for a few seconds.

2. Repeat all four movements once again.

3. Repeat with the left shoulder.

Helpful Hint: Don't worry if you hear crackling sounds —it's only natural.

▬ Shake Away ⊽

For: Loosening hands and wrists

Where: Sitting on the bed, or anywhere
Here's one sure way to stimulate the circulation when your fingers fall asleep.

Preparation: Lift up your right hand and let it hang limp as though it were falling off the wrist.
1. Shake it rapidly for at least ten seconds as though it were wet and you were drying it. Continue shaking until hand feels rubbery.
2. Now do the same with the left hand.

ON-THE-SPOT RELAXERS

We can all learn from plant life that there are times for growth and times for rest. The body needs time to slow down at least once a day whether it's because of pressures brought home from the office, or just family chores. Since total relaxation is often impossible to achieve during a busy day, be kind to yourself and learn to compensate. As someone once said, "Pleasant relaxation opens the way for a flow of energy and strength." Here are a few exercises to relax you when you want to unwind completely. Try one or two, and repeat them whenever tension gets you down.

▬ Meltaway

This is one of my favorites and one I've used many times in teaching. You should be lying down on the floor, but it can always be adapted to a reclining or sitting position. Try it once and you'll want to do it again and again.

Lie down on any comfortable surface. Stretch out on your back with your arms out to the sides, palms down, legs slightly apart.

Close your eyes, open your lips slightly to relax the jaw, and shut out all thoughts except those of self. Imagine you are alone on a soft, sandy beach where all you can hear are the sounds of waves gently caressing the shore. Feel the glow of the hot sun pouring down on your body and then try to feel your limbs and every part of torso melting away as though made of wax. Begin with the feet, and focusing on one area at a time, feel each part of you gradually become soft and limp, released of all energy. When your thoughts focus on your face, feel as though your eyes, nose, and mouth are becoming soft and motionless. Finally let go—and feel yourself melt away into the sand.

▬▬ Burst the Balloon

Sit in a chair and close your eyes, dropping your head to your chest. Breathe in letting your head lift slightly, then breathe out by blowing the air slowly and as you do so, feel as though your body were a balloon; as you release the air, the balloon deflates and your head and torso drop toward the ground.

▬▬ Instant Lower Back Relaxer ⊻

Pinch in the derrière and hold for a few seconds. Now relax and let go. Repeat at least eight times. Each time the derrière muscles tighten, they will automatically release some tension in the lower back. This exercise is particularly useful if you have to stand on your feet all day.

▬▬ Overall Relaxer ⊻

One way of letting go of tension in the body is to think of the puppet again. Imagine that a string was lifting up your shoulder, hand, or leg, and that then suddenly the string snapped and your shoulder, hand, or leg dropped lifeless. It's not always so easy to let go like this, but when you're very tense, it is important that you try. So practice it a few times until you learn to really "let go!"

5

Shower Power
–Wherever You Go!

THE MINI-SERIES

If you can't squeeze more than a few exercises into your daily routine, let me suggest that you create your own mini-series of exercises by selecting from those already described before in the chapters on the bath and shower, and après bath and shower. Look through them all and decide which ones will benefit you most. Include in your mini-series a few from the shower or bath and one all-purpose exercise from the towel series.

It is always important to do the exercises as part of your bath or shower routine, since it is the warm water that makes all the difference to your muscles and the flexibility of your spine. However, there is no reason why you shouldn't take the exercises along with you to the office, on vacation, or wherever you go. In a sense, your mini-series constitutes the cream of the crop—exercises that are as essential to a beautiful and healthy body as cleansing itself.

For an effective and complete body stretch, do at least EIGHT exercises chosen from the following list. No matter which you select, try to include a Neck/Shoulder Stretch, the Supine Pelvic Tilt, and a Hamstring Stretch. These are crucial for loosening the back muscles and maintaining suppleness.

From the Shower Series
Head Rotations
Shoulder Rotations
Waist Twist
Pelvic Roll

From the Bath Series
Head Rotations
Shoulder Rotations
Torso Twist
Forward Bend
Knee and Ankle Hug

From the Après Shower and Bath Series
Pelvic Tilt—Rib Cage Lift
Leg Stretch
The Big O
Body Roll

SPOT WARM-UPS

Here's a good warm-up routine that you can do in just a few seconds to loosen back muscles; take it slowly!

Head: Draw an oval with your nose

Shoulders: Draw circles with the shoulders

Waist: Twist the upper torso from side to side without moving the pelvis

Pelvis: Tilt pelvis in one fluid movement; then circle hips

To loosen tight upper back muscles: Shoulder Rotations, Angel Wings, Backstroke

To loosen tight lower back muscles: Derrière Pinch-Hold-Release, Pelvic Tilt, Knee and Ankle Hug.

To loosen the entire back: Bend Over—Roll Up with or without towel, Body Roll.

A PLAN FOR DYNAMIC POSTURE

From the beginning of this book I have focused on the abdominal muscles because I have seen so many women discouraged by what are often futile attempts to maintain a flat tummy and firm derrière. They have heard "Hold in your stomach!" or "Stand up straight," as if just pressing a magic button would make those things happen. Pinch-pull-elongate *will* keep your stomach flat and your derrière firm, BUT it must become a way of life rather than just an occasional exercise.

In addition to the exercises described, you may want to work on a program that will *insure* good posture and strong, firm abdominals. For this reason, I have outlined a suggested plan. Take these steps one at a time. Remember: One must learn to crawl before walking.

Step 1:

Building Strong Abdominals with Held Contractions and Rhythmic Breathing

1. Begin with the Mini-Sit-Ups (Chapter 4); do them at least twice a day. Try to hold the contraction as long as possible without getting neck tension. Aim for at least six mini-sit-ups, then relax completely.

2. Repeat the pinch-pull-elongate action at least three times before & after bathing. Hold the contraction for as long as possible, aiming for a count of eight to twelve.

3. Repeat the Supine Pelvic Tilt and Rib Cage Lift daily—with rhytmic breathing.

Step 2:

Activating Abdominal Muscles in Steady Partial Contraction, Breathing Normally

1. Repeat the Pelvic Tilt (or Pelvic Roll) with your bath or shower.

2. Whenever you are standing in one place—waiting at a counter, talking on the phone—think pinch pull, elongate!

3. Write out the words *pinch* and *pull* and paste them on the bathroom mirror, refrigerator, desk, and over the visor of the car, to remind yourself to keep those muscles working!

4. Whenever you get a chance to look at yourself in the mirror, think "elongation." Hold that elongated posture as though someone were taking your picture. With your rib cage lifted, notice how much slimmer your waist is!

When you are moving about, think Dynamic Posture; that means activating the abdominal muscles. Here are some golden opportunities for doing so:

Whenever you are involved in a walking activity, elongate your back and think pinch and pull (there are endless possibilities for this on a hike or on the golf course).

During active sports, whenever you have to take a break—on the ski lift, tennis court, or in the bowling alley—think pinch and pull.

As you are building up abdominal tone, your muscles will begin to work naturally. Without your even being aware, they will respond as an involuntary action. When that glorious moment comes, you will have achieved Dynamic Posture!

One of the best ways to get into the Dynamic Posture habit is to include it with daily walking. Walking contains all the ingredients that are so beneficial to beauty and health—good posture, stretching, proper breathing, mental relaxation, and freedom of movement in the arms and legs. And walking with authority brings movement to form. When the form (or figure) is correctly aligned, and the movement free, easy, and brisk, walking becomes an exercise that both clears the mind and conditions the body. When performed at a rapid pace, it controls weight and builds stamina. Did you know that you burn almost as many calories walking a mile as you do running a mile?

Walking as an exercise means walking briskly as opposed to sauntering. It is moving at a rhythmic pace—whatever is comfortable for your body—with arms relaxed, so there is no tension in your shoulders or upper back, and feet moving directly forward. There is a certain amount of productive effort to bring all the correct muscles into play, and that, of course, is good for your shape. Above all, walking is the only exercise that you can do virtually anywhere. If you want to get even more exercise from a walk, include walking up and down some hills or climbing stairs steadily—good for the heart, the legs, and for building endurance. Don't take walking for granted. Bring a friend along for company and do it regularly.

If you want to lose a bit of weight or build up more muscle tone, you can increase your walking pace until you are almost jogging. Begin by walking a mile at a brisk but comfortable pace, then increase the pace till you are doing about three miles an hour. Jogging should be done under a doctor's supervision and, when possible, on a track-type surface.

Today more and more women are participating in various active sports not just for health purposes, but for recreation. For any woman who wants to select activities that are particularly beneficial for the figure, let me give you my personal favorites. As a dancer I am partial to any activity that develops abdominal muscle tone, tightens leg muscles, and keeps the body flexible and supple. Brisk walking, swimming, and dancing—three of my favorites—are all great for women of any age. They are not only invigorating but are as wonderful for the psyche as they are for all-purpose conditioning.

Regardless of your personal taste, try to get involved in at least one sport activity and stick with it. And I hope you will always remember to prepare your muscles first with the warm water workouts! You will notice a considerable difference in performance when you do, especially in cold or damp weather. The ballet dancer depends on at least a half hour of warm-ups at the barre and a leotard, tights, and/or leg warmers to protect the muscles and keep them warmed. Dr. Hans Kraus, who has worked with countless numbers of dancers and teachers, has said, "You don't take a horse out of the stable and run him like mad before warming him up." What many people don't realize is that preparing muscles for active sports means bending, stretching, flexing—not merely pregame practicing!

Today's woman has every opportunity to be creative and productive in so many areas. She is achieving both when she can meet the challenge and, despite her years, maintain an attractive, youthful figure and a feeling of vitality. I hope Shower Power can contribute to it.

As you enter your private spa, and whenever you leave it, remember that the name of the game is relaxing and stretching. It is what your muscles beg for—so treat them with extra loving care.

Whether you are sixteen or sixty, slim or overweight, be kind to yourself and take some time each day to relax, reshape, and revitalize. Shower Power is the way to give yourself two of life's most precious gifts—a more youthful, attractive figure *and* the flexibility and freedom of movement that you knew as a child and can recapture as an adult.